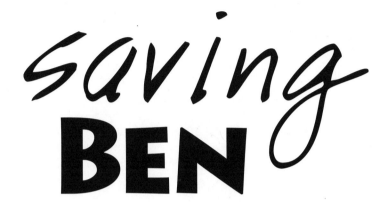

saving BEN

A Father's Story of Autism

DAN E. BURNS

Number 3 in the Mayborn Literary Nonfiction Series

University of North Texas Press
Mayborn Graduate Institute of Journalism
Denton, Texas

Permissions:
University of North Texas Press
1155 Union Circle #311336
Denton, TX 76203-5017

The paper used in this book meets the minimum requirements of the American National Standard for Permanence of Paper for Printed Library Materials, z39.48.1984. Binding materials have been chosen for durability.

Library of Congress Cataloging-in-Publication Data

Burns, Dan E. (Dan Eric), 1945–
  Saving Ben : a father's story of autism / by Dan E. Burns. — 1st ed.
    p. cm. — (Mayborn literary nonfiction series ; no. 3)
  ISBN 978-1-57441-269-7 (cloth : alk. paper)
    1. Burns, Dan E. (Dan Eric), 1945– . 2. Burns, Ben, 1987– . 3. Parents of autistic children—Texas—Biography. 4. Autistic children—Texas—Biography. 5. Autistic youth—Texas—Biography. 6. Fathers and sons—Texas—Biography. 7. Autism—Texas. I. Title. II. Series: Mayborn literary nonfiction series ; no. 3.
  RC553.A88B87   2009
  362.198'928588200922—dc22
  [B]
                                                                    2009010163

Saving Ben: A Father's Story of Autism is Number 3 in the Mayborn Literary Nonfiction Series

Interior design by Joseph Parenteau.

To all my children

CONTENTS

PREFACE

This is not the book I had hoped to write. Soon after Ben was diagnosed in 1990, I began keeping a diary. By 1995 I had accumulated more than five hundred pages of observations, fears, and hopes, all shaped by the vision that someday he would emerge from autism and re-enter the world practically indistinguishable from someone who had never been afflicted. Indeed, hundreds if not thousands of preschool children are recovering from autism (see www.autism. com), and I still hold onto the hope that someday, Ben will be among them. But by 2008, when he turned twenty-one, "someday" had crossed the river to a more perfect time and place where every tear will be wiped away. Until then I have an imperfect story of an ongoing struggle, one that has left me with much to celebrate, and much to grieve.

This book is in a sense an answer to my grief. When I sat down in December of 2007 and wrote the first sentence, I could not have said how the book would end, or even why I was writing it. I only knew that the time had come. I dreaded writing the scenes that exposed aspects of myself I would have preferred to keep hidden, but it became clear to me as I relived those times that Ben's story was inseparable from his mother's story and from my own. Autistic children discover the fault lines in a marriage, and their fates hinge on challenges to the family, how we rise or fall: how we resolve our guilt, our anger, our shame; how we reach out to a future that seems at times dark as the Styx. Perhaps I could help other parents struggling with autism and with the medical profession, the school system, their marriages, and themselves. I had only to tell the truth.

In the end, I found that I had written a recovery story after all. What is recovered is a family more resilient, forgiving, and loving. Like the characters in *The Wizard of Oz*, we have made a journey through a perilous land, and we have discovered in ourselves the gifts that prepare us to seek the future beyond the fear, the darkness. After the earthquake, wind, and fire, a still, small voice of peace.

The journey is not mine alone. It is yours, brave, brokenhearted father and mother; it is yours, teacher, doctor, preacher, caregiver, administrator, scientist, politician, you who see in the tragedy and triumph of a child a challenge and a hope. We do not know why some children recover and others do not. We have much to learn about autism etiologies and effective treatments. At the end of the road is not a gleaming emerald city, but a promise: We will persevere. We will tell our stories. We shall continue our journey. Together, we will overcome.

Acknowledgments

I am indebted to the many professionals and family members who walked beside me on this healing journey: To Dr. Bernard Rimland, who established *Defeat Autism Now!* and pioneered the behavioral and the biomedical treatments that are helping so many children. His personal response to my queries nudged me in the right direction. To Dr. Constantine Kotsanis, who helped pioneer the new biomedical protocols. He gave Ben's mom and me valuable professional advice when most conventionally trained doctors offered no treatment and no hope. To Sharon Hawkins, Ben's aide and "mom-at-school," who took him into her heart and home during the darkest days. To the Reverend Shelley A. Hamilton, for her prayers these many years. To Mom, who was always there when Ben and I needed her, who still speaks in the spirit of love whispering through these pages. To Ben's mom, Susan, who with courage and persistence overcame her crippling psychological disorder to help revive Ben's biomedical program. To Ben, my courageous, wonderful son.

I am also indebted to the writers, critics, and editors who helped me construct a coherent, well-paced narrative: To Sandra Williams, Ph.D., whose quick and cogent feedback helped shape every scene, whose encouragement and admonishments kept me writing through long months when the task seemed endless. To Mark Noble and the gang at The Writer's Garret peer workshop, Stone Soup, who provided useful technical feedback and cheered me on. To my senior editor, Ronald Chrisman, whose steady hand guided the manuscript through many drafts. To George Getschow, writer-in-residence of the Mayborn Conference, whose reading, editing, and invigorating questions prompted a cover-to-cover rewrite, and to the farsighted folks at the Mayborn Graduate School of Journalism, whose award made this book possible.

Thank you.

PART 1

THE STORM

WISHED UPON A STAR

July 1990. Carrollton, Texas

The Carrollton Public Library didn't smell like an office; it smelled of cedar pencil shavings and Windex, an elementary school classroom. The tables were populated by schoolchildren writing their book reports. I was dressed for success: suit, tie, and briefcase. I didn't belong here. Likely a pedophile, the librarian no doubt thought, playing hooky from work.

I should be in an office building downtown, handing speech drafts to a secretary, or on an American Airlines flight to New York to interview the CEO of IBM, or giving a presentation in the Dell boardroom.

The librarian, black-frocked Miss Colfin, hair done up in a Pentecostal bun, pretended to ignore me but I felt she was watching out of the corner of her eye. Would she think I was going to stash books in my briefcase and sneak out? Would she think it was full of drugs?

Trying to look professional, I found the card catalogue and pulled out the musty "AU" drawer.

"No, Blunderbuss," a voice in my head said, addressing me.

One of my inner characters was afraid that Miss Colfin might put two and two together and deduce that I was searching for books on autism. "The pedophile must have an autistic son," she would surmise.

And that would make Ben autistic.

Turning my back on Miss Colfin to shield the file drawer from her view, I thumbed through the cards. There was only one book on autism, and the title was not reassuring: *The Ultimate Stranger.*

I pulled the book from the shelves, found a secluded table, and flipped through the pages.

"Endlessly biting his own hand, screaming like a wounded animal when you approach, endlessly slapping his own face, finger-painting his body with his own feces … this is the autistic child," wrote Carl H. Delacato, the author.

If had been in the bathroom I'd have thrown up. I saw myself straddling the space between the washbasins, looking in the mirror. "This is not me," I would have thought, hands trembling. "Not me furtively scouring the back shelves of a public library at two-thirty in the afternoon, not me with baby puke on my suit, red-eyed, wrinkled, and unkempt. I've wandered off the set of the movie they are making about my life and stumbled into somebody else's film."

This is not me any more than the children described in this accursed book are like my three-year-old son.

Sometime in the dim and distant past, distracted by grief, I'd turned my old gray Buick left in front of speeding motorcycle. The bike hit the passenger door, flipping the rider over the top of the car. This is not happening, I thought. And for a moment I believed it.

Whew. That was a close one. For a minute there I almost thought—ha ha—Ben was autistic. Silly Dad. He's as normal as you or me, just slow, like Grandma and Grandpa said.

Boom. And the body hit the ground.

I stashed the book in my briefcase and fled.

🐸   🐸   🐸

Three years earlier …

"Scissors." *Snip.*

"Big head," said the doctor. And out came Benjamin, my third child, beloved son. Sue went into false labor on the Fourth of July, 1987, and from the hospital window we could see bursts of fireworks branding the sky, followed by the tardy pa-pa-pa-pop that sounded like champagne corks toasting Ben's arrival. Though his birth was delayed until the middle of August, he was to be my fireworks baby, inheritor of everything his siblings had missed. At a party to celebrate Midsummer's Eve I explained to a former professor, a nun who specialized in Emily Dickinson, that Ben's brother and sister had grown up with hand-me-down clothes and Salvation Army bikes. But with my new job as the speechwriter for the CEO of a major oil company and an empty nest, "We can afford to give Benjamin whatever he wants."

The nun was unimpressed. She took a sip of her wine. "Don't," she said, "spoil him."

But I was looking forward to spoiling him. Ten years of penury in Stillwater, Oklahoma, living hand to mouth on graduate school stipends and my wife's salary, had given me an itch for a life without fear of overdrafts, a life lulled by the sturdy and certain flap-flap-flap of the cash machine. In the 1980s, oil-rich Dallas, J. R. Ewing's boomtown, was the ultimate cash machine. Sue and I were dressed for success, an image from *Ozzie and Harriet.* "That necklace Harriet wore?" said Sue. "I want one like it. Those are Republican pearls."

Surely no child has ever been more eagerly anticipated than Benjamin. "Don't you want a sweet little baby?" said Sue, in bed, the night he was conceived, her hand seeking an answer. "A sweet, itty-bitty baby?" I said no, but looking out the window that clear cold January evening at a twinkling star, I wished upon it, and we rolled the dice. Yes, I wanted another baby. I wanted another chance to be a great dad.

      ❧   ❧   ❧

1962. Stillwater, Oklahoma

The first time Susan moved from the fringes of my conscious-
ness to somewhere near the center, she was in my way. She sat one
desk ahead of me in high school geometry, junior year.

Two minutes until the 12:50 bell. I could feel the lunch line
lengthening. Mr. Mihura, the teacher, was droning on and on about
point Q at the intersection of a ray that bisects parallel blah, blah,
one minute until the bell. Susan raised her hand and Mihura was
driving into overtime for sure.

"Mr. Mihura?"

"Shut up," I hissed.

Susan turned around and stared at me. She was the only girl I
knew who wore sunglasses indoors.

"Lunch," I stage-whispered, pointing to the clock.

"Tough titty."

The bell rang and Susan was up and out of her desk, blocking
the aisle, jamming books and papers into satchels that hung off her
body like overstuffed butt cheeks, half the students already out the
door. "Class dismissed," said Mihura. Susan lurched into the aisle
in front of me, swinging her ass, a moving obstacle blocking the
fast lane. I was hungry for lunch, impatient, and to my seventeen-
year-old eyes she looked like a granny driver in a '53 Ford pickup,
going twenty miles an hour in a high-speed zone, me stuck in traffic
behind her. I imagined her driving a beat-up truck farting black ex-
haust, blocking my way as I tried to pass to the right or the left, her
book satchels bouncing off her hips like piles of sandbags rocking
and rolling off the tailgate.

That was the year I told Dad that I was gay. "No, you're not,"
he argued. "You just need to meet the right girl." In search of Miss
Right, I gave a party for my friends but only a few came. After the
last goodnights were said, Susan stood beside me.

"Let's laugh," she urged. "Let's laugh for one minute."

I held my watch up and we *aha-ha-ha*'d as loud as we could, kept
it going. But I couldn't tell from looking at Susan's face whether she

was laughing or crying. There in the deserted living room, lights low, music playing, she looked up and put her mouth to mine. "Thy breath was shed / Upon my soul between the kisses and the wine," wrote Ernest Dowson. Now I understood. I was smitten.

Next day Susan and I skipped study hall and snuck to the brook. Waving her wand, she summoned up the creek snakes. Heads poked out of the water like little Loch Ness monsters. "I want to paint you naked," she told me. That night, after *David and Lisa*, a movie about star-crossed teenage lovers, I pulled up in her driveway. I was kissing her goodnight when her tongue took me by surprise. I accidentally stepped on the accelerator and smashed Mom's T-Bird through the garage door.

Reined in by the adults in her family, devalued—"You never *were* worth the trouble," said her mother—Susan saw herself as Cinderella sitting among the clinkers. Her self-portraits showed hard, bony figures with swollen, outsized hands and knuckles, drooping faces, waiting. Her favorite tune was Miles Davis's haunting trumpet solo, "Someday My Prince Will Come."

Enchanted, I fancied myself her prince. The Age of Aquarius was dawning, and Susan was an Aquarian, bound to the wellsprings of art, music, literature. In my adolescent mind, awash in hyperbole and hormones, all compasses pointed toward her. Tides moved with her moods. Subterranean rivers flowed through her veins. Blossoms opened and closed as she passed, and moon vines bred in her footsteps, flowers with fresh white faces lifted, like hers, toward the sky.

My boyfriend was Joel, a year older, my guide to all that was dark and dangerous, serpent in my Garden of Eden. Tennessee Williams once had picked sixteen-year-old Joel out of a line of boys and men hustling sex in Fayetteville, Arkansas. Williams said Joel looked literary, and Joel took the compliment to heart. His ambition was to become a bestselling author, like Jack Kerouac. There in the Moonlight Lounge by the drive-in theater, he assumed his *Rebel Without a Cause* pose, sleeves rolled up like an arm wrestler, and drummed his left-hand fingers on the table to a beat only he could hear: drummed and moved his head and shoulders side to side like a cobra. Joel believed that anyone of either gender who looked into his unblinking eyes would fall in love with him.

"Stillwater. Armpit of the world," he said. He licked his lips and blew onto his shoulder, a wet fart.

So it went: Joel by night, Susan by day.

Every weekday I would pick Susan up at 7:15 a.m., drive her to school, leave my Model A with the "Goldwater for President" sticker in the parking lot. After school we'd meet at the car and I would drive her to the Campus Drugstore and buy her an ice cream.

One Friday afternoon I found Susan wandering around the parking lot. The Model A wasn't where we'd left it that morning.

"Where did you go?" she asked.

"Joel and I went to DeLavon's for lunch."

Her green eyes flashed. Like a Rottweiler that turns on a kid, no warning, she fast-slapped me. "Princess was always such a good dog," says the bewildered owner, "a good dog."

In the end, I married the Rottweiler.

❧   ❧   ❧

July 1967. Iowa City, Iowa

Clearly, I had found the right girl. Sue believed in fairy-tale endings, and when it came right down to it, so did I. But marriage didn't make me straight. Shortly after Susan and I settled into our new home in Iowa City, a former army barracks converted to married student housing, a maintenance worker arrived to paint the window trim green. Looking out the bedroom window, I watched him from the bed where Sue and I had recently finished celebrating our marital privileges. He was young, cute, and shirtless. My mind said no but my dick didn't get the message.

"Oh shit," I thought. "I'm still gay."

Here I was with a child on the way, married to a dependent wife whom I had promised to love, honor, and obey. Yet I couldn't keep my eyes off that shirtless painter.

I remembered Dad's advice when I confessed my inclinations to him: "Put a lid on it, put it in a safe, take it down to the basement, dig a deep hole, and pour concrete on it."

That's what I did. For the next twenty-five years, I became the person I thought Mom and Dad wanted me to be: the successful, upwardly mobile Dr. Jekyll. My heterosexual persona became a suit of armor, a shell that defended me from the outside world. But there was another person hiding deep inside. And if the lid came off every so often and Mr. Hyde came out for a romp, who was to know, and what harm was done?

Quirky Ben

August 1987. Carrollton, Texas

"**D**o you think the hospital would take him back?" I asked Sue in mock exasperation.

"We could leave him on the steps," she kidded. We both laughed and welcomed the comic relief. After two days of Ben at home we were exhausted. He screamed. Before feeding, after feeding, while his diaper was changed, bedtime to witching hour, Ben screeched like a madman howling through a megaphone. Twenty minutes of sleep, more screeching, another short nap if we were lucky, then back to the megaphone. Our other two kids hadn't been like this.

But Ben wasn't like our other kids; no, not from hour zero. First, his head was gigantic, above the 98th percentile, off the charts, sticking out of his mom's birth canal then out of the papoose wrapper like a preposterous Tootsie Roll Pop. I held my newborn son while the doctor sewed up Sue. *Big head,* I thought, *good. With all that space for brains, he'll be a genius.* But as the medics wheeled him down the hall, he screeched woefully, painfully.

"Stop," I yelled. They stopped the cart. "Something hurts," I insisted, rushing up to Ben. Could it be a wayward safety pin?

"No," the medics assured me, the first of many lies doctors would tell us about our son. "He's OK."

OK? Then why is he screaming?

"We don't know," they might as well have said, "it's not our job."

Then whose job is it? Surely not … mine?

At home, Ben didn't take the teat. He lost weight, failed to thrive. He lay at the bottom of the baby bag, a kangaroo pouch, emaciated, a concentration camp victim.

At the pediatrician's urging we switched from breast milk to baby formula, Enfamil, loads of which he burped up or projectile-vomited. "I know how much you love our son," Sue explained. "I wanted to breast-feed him because I thought it would make you love me more." We walked around the kitchen and nursery with towels on our shoulders, ready for the next Enfamil moment. But the formula that stayed down seemed to nourish him. Ben gained weight, though his head was growing faster than his body. And he screamed and screamed. "It's colic," the doctor assured us. "He'll outgrow it."

Our older children were busy with their own lives. Hannah was a senior in high school, working at Target, miffed by this usurper who took her place as the youngest child in the family, worried that people would think Ben was her baby. Pete was living in his own apartment, coming home weekends to practice with his garage band, which drowned Ben's cries. We learned to cope.

Ben loved to be held and rocked, but for the worst of his gut storms the rocking chair wasn't enough. I bounced him up and down on the bed: the bigger the bounce, the better. I put him in the baby carriage and raced him over the roughest parts of the side-walk. I drove him around in the back seat, seeking bumpier roads. I set him on top of the washing machine and juiced it up to the spin cycle. I took him horseback riding, swung him in his baby bag, tossed him high, high, higher. Ben would squeal his joy, then burp, leaking Enfamil. The burp signaled a few minutes of peace.

On the sunny side, Ben loved music and kinetic nursery rhymes. He'd squeal with delight at action-packed thrillers—Jack *jump* over the candlestick, Wee Willy Winkie *runs* through the town, Scotland's burning: Fire, fire, fire. He'd jam his palms together, clapping, and demand encore after encore. He craved to be knee-bounced on the rhyming words: "One, two, buckle my *shoe*. Three, four, close the *door.*" His favorite games were hide and seek and "Here comes the big hairy monster: *Arrrrgh.*" Tickle tickle tickle *squeal.* Followed by the blessed Enfamil burp.

Ben preferred looking at things and people upside down. He'd hang backwards over a cushion or pillow, his arched back a U-turn, his head an inverted smiley face, and he'd lock his radar-detector gaze onto my eyes. "Look," said my brother, Cris, sitting across the room with Mom and Dad. "They're bonding." And indeed we were. Gazing into Ben's eyes, I felt a connection so deep that I had to give voice to it. "I will always love you," I said. "I will never, never abandon you." It was a vow I would keep in times better and worse.

🐌   🐌   🐌

November 1987. Dallas, Texas

By the time Ben was three months old, Sue was receiving urgent phone calls from her boss urging her to cut her leave of absence short and return to work. Or else.

"Dan," Sue asked me, "Can you take care of Benjamin *and* the business?"

I thought about it. Well, I was already working at home, marketing my speechwriting software, *Thoughtline.* My start-up business produced cash flow, but Sue's job with the Dallas Park and Recreation Department paid for the medical insurance that funded our high-maintenance baby. Raising a baby and a business together would be difficult, but I was a Burns, following in the footsteps of my entrepreneurial father, whose business card read "Difficult tasks performed immediately. The impossible may take a little longer." Hadn't I organized a commune of Canadian hippies into a documentary film production company? Hadn't I landed one great job after another, taught myself software engineering, created an innovative speechwriting product, and launched my own company?

"You bet," I answered.

"Great," said Sue. And she was gone.

I'd had a preschool playhouse and had learned to cook waffles and beat eggs, but my domestic training was cut short when I was arrested—yanked out by the collar—for playing in the girls' sandbox at school. It had more sand. Except for vegetables wrapped in tinfoil and tossed in the campfire, a culinary skill I'd learned as a Boy Scout, food was something set in front of me by a mother, grandmother, or school cafeteria lunch lady. As I grew older I understood that there were various theories of nutrition troubling the land, and my position was that diets were like religion: matters of personal belief, numerous and contradictory; they could not be proved or disproved and had no practical application for me. My weight stayed forty pounds below the boiling point of water and was just about as invariable.

My entrepreneurial training, however, was outstanding. In fifth grade my best friend, Scrib, and I invested in a squeegee and set up a regular window-washing route along Main Street. We fancied ourselves the Wright Brothers. We designed fantastic flying machines and built a motorized go-cart, attracting the attention—and cash commissions—of neighborhood children who wanted a go-cart like ours.

On the one hand I was well prepared to grow a home-based software business. On the other, I was only marginally prepared to assume primary care for a high-maintenance child like Ben.

"What happens," Dad used to ask, "when an irresistible force meets an immovable object?" The question was supposed to be a stumper, but in the real world when continents collide—the one immovable, the other irresistible—a mountain range arises. The mountain range was the altered landscape of my life, challenging as Everest.

Not every day was equally challenging. On good days, four-month-old Ben was an easy baby. He'd sit strapped in his seat on the shipping desk and study his mobile while I staffed the communications desk a few feet away. I'd be lost in my work for an hour or so, then I'd notice that Ben was still mesmerized by the mobile. Shouldn't I be stimulating him? Odd, I thought, but my motto was Do Not Disturb a Quiet Baby.

For a change of venue I'd take Ben downstairs and set him in his baby swing in front of the television. His favorite shows were *Wheel of Fortune*—he loved the spinning and clapping—and *The Weather Channel*, which in those days consisted of a radar scan line sweeping around Texas at the approximate speed of a minute hand, the most boring broadcast on TV. Ben loved it. "It's slow," said Sue, "like him."

For a rainy day diversion, Sue tied a mailing tube to the rocking chair. Ben would drop a walnut down the tube and listen, watching while it rolled to the other end. Fascinated, he'd pick up the walnut and do it again until we distracted him. I pictured him as a patient scientist performing an experiment over and over until he got every last bit of information. Couldn't he roll something else down the tube, a marble, a wooden bead? No, had to be a walnut. Such intense concentration. He'd be a research scientist, or an engineer. Such persistence. Such dedication. Such single-mindedness. Surely these were the qualities of an Edison.

Like Edison, Ben had ear infections and colic. On difficult days he cried inconsolably. Mom, who handled a good chunk of the babysitting, told me the story of her phone call to Dr. Neal, my pediatrician. "Danny won't stop crying. What can I do?" she asked.

"Go to the drugstore and pick up a prescription of phenobarbital, a bottle of whiskey, and a shot glass," the good doctor answered.

"You want me to give my baby whiskey?"

"Give him the phenobarbital. Then pour yourself a shot of whiskey."

I could sympathize with Mom. There are few things worse than being unable to help a child in pain. On the bright side, though, colic is caused by a buildup of gas pressure in leaky intestines like overpressurized steam in an ancient rusty boiler—safety valves hissing, alarms ringing, needles in the red zone—the baby never explodes, though sometimes the parent may. Eventually the crisis subsides, though never, as any survivor will tell you, soon enough.

❧   ❧   ❧

The ear infections began crowding one on top of another about age one. Sue and I set Ben on the bed, his forehead hot as the orange bedspread, fever spiking.

"This is scaring me, Dan."

"Let's go."

It was the first of many late-night trips to the Kaiser HMO emergency room, all following the same script: the sudden shrieks of pain late at night or in the wee hours of the morning, the frightened drive through darkness, the long wait in the comfortless fluorescent room whose bare walls echoed Ben's screams, the prescription for pink bubblegum-flavored Amoxicillin that Ben would spit out all over his clothes and us. We mixed it with applesauce or squirted it down his gullet with a turkey baster. He threw up so much of it we often had to order a refill: a ten-day prescription lasted only about a week. We hoped that we got enough of it down him to do some good.

Ben would improve for a couple of weeks until he was knocked down with another ear infection, which would be treated exactly as if it were the first. Ben's doctors—or "service providers," as the Kaiser Permanente HMO preferred to call them—simply followed the medical algorithm, the repair manual. When I pointed out that Ben's ear infections were recurrent, six in four months, I thought the medical service provider would say, "Yes, you are right. What is driving these infections? Let's get to the bottom of it." That didn't happen. So we added another bottle of gooey Amoxicillin to the collection in the fridge. Perhaps some other doctor could have helped, but with limited finances we felt that we were stuck, for insurance purposes, in the Kaiser-Permanente system.

A dozen years later I sit in my study, going through Ben's medical records from 1987 through 1991. I turn the tattered pages of these fading carbon copies, these pink and yellow forms. It takes the better part an afternoon to read through them. Some nearly illegible, but it doesn't matter, because they nearly all say the same thing: "Acute distress ... child crying *hard* ... pulling at right ear ... thrush on tongue and throat ... yellow mucus ... inflammation ... passing gas ... diarrhea ... severe diaper rash ...screaming and kicking ... vomiting." Further, the treatment was always the same, more antibiotics: Amoxicillin, Ceclor, Septra.

I count 173 records of visits to the Kaiser emergency room, Ben's Kaiser pediatrician Dr. Eakman, a referred specialist, or to a lab, between Ben's first birthday, when the ear infections started in earnest, and Ben's fourth birthday, when he received his four-year vaccinations and began the last leg of his descent.

One hundred and seventy-three medical events in three years.

The last time I saw poor, hapless Dr. Eakman, he excused himself from the medical examination room and was gone for so long that I went looking for him. I found him in an office, sitting at a desk, reading a thick red book—the *Physicians' Desk Reference.* I hadn't thought of it until then, but likely Dr. Eakman was as frustrated in his own way as Sue and I were. The answers we needed were not in the book. A few weeks later Eakman resigned from clinical practice to go back to school so he could pursue a career in medical research. I wished him the best. I might have quit too if I'd known where to submit my resignation.

& & &

As Ben approached his developmental milestones we were with him every step of the way, helping. We taught him how to hold a bottle, how to roll over, how to pull up his blanket, crawl, sit up, stand up, walk. It wasn't that Ben couldn't move his limbs; it was that he seemed surprised that they were attached to his body: he didn't know what to do with them. So we showed him by moving them for him. We were the puppeteers and he was the puppet. To teach him to crawl we pushed him across the rug while we puppeteered his arms and legs. To teach him to walk, we coaxed year-old Ben to fall forward into my arms while his mom bike-pedaled his legs to keep them under him.

Ben learned to scramble up anything. He would climb out of any crib, escape from any playpen. Turn around and we were likely to find him on the table or the kitchen cabinet. He'd have mounted the refrigerator if he could have found a foothold.

To our eyes, all of this odd behavior was endearingly quirky. How else to explain our indulgence of his obsessions? He'd collect long, straight, pointed objects—sticks or soda straws, coat hangers, long stems of grass—which he squirreled away in odd nooks. He'd run about the house bouncing from wall to wall and waving these objects a few feet in front of his face yelling *E-e-e-e-e* like a daredevil, a kamikaze pilot, Evel Knievel performing his Grand Canyon jump. How charming. How precocious.

Running and screeching constituted his routine during the day. But at night? Ben didn't distinguish between sunrise and sunset. Every night was a lock-in party, a contest to see who could stay awake the longest. Ben always won. While his stuporous parents tried to sleep, Ben walked around the house on the balls of his feet, toes curled under, waving his wire coat hanger, sucking his bottle, mustering Mom and Dad to demand a refill, another hit of Enfamil. Next morning we'd find him passed out on the floor beside his crib, diapers yellow, heavy, and stinking of ammonia, or curled up in the fireplace pit, or on the couch, or in his sister's clothes closet, or in the nook under the stairs.

He chewed his wet diapers. He flipped light switches on and off. He raided the coin jar and filled his mouth with pennies and nickels. He ate with his fingers and wiped his hands on the walls. Then there was the grape raid ritual. Ben would sneak a purple grape from the fruit bowl and beeline to the nearest exit, a shoplifter fleeing the cops, legs spinning like the Looney Tunes roadrunner as he stuffed the pilfered grape into his mouth. Halfway to the door he'd stop short and stare at his empty hand as if in disbelief, Marcel Marceau miming comic surprise: *Where's the grape?* Then he'd turn around, spy the fruit—*Aha!*—and trot resolutely back to filch another purple prize. "His feet work faster than his brain," quipped Uncle Tever.

Ben also was becoming more sensitive to sounds.

"Attention, Kmart shoppers," barked the voice from the overhead speaker. "Blue Light Special on aisle five."

Ben covered his ears, screamed and scrambled for the exit as if pursued by the four trampling horsemen of the Apocalypse. His face—Munch's *The Scream* looked comic by comparison—testified to his terror. His pediatrician ordered a brain stem audio test. All of Ben's auditory equipment was working normally. What was I worried about?

Well, for one thing, some days Ben was as slow as a gravel truck climbing a mountain.

"Throw it, throw it," I called to Ben from the bottom of the staircase. He was on the landing at the middle holding a heavy orange rubber ball pitted like a moon rock. It had been a carefully chosen first birthday present, something we could play with together. From his perch on the stairs he'd give a toss and bouncy, bouncy, bouncy, *boom*. Down it would roll. He'd squeal with delight as I tossed it again and again, playing fetch with tireless Rover. But our playtimes, it seemed, were becoming few and shorter. Sue and I assumed that once Ben had learned a behavior, leaned how to hold a pencil, draw a line, say a word, untie and remove his shoe, that he'd learned it for all time and would move on. But we were wrong. Yesterday he could take off his shoe; today he can't, or won't. It is raining, the guests will arrive in twenty minutes, I am out of coffee and must take Ben to the store with me. But he has forgotten how to put on his shiny yellow rain boots. I put them on for him just this one time. I discover that this one time becomes every time.

Today I'd had enough. My eighteen-month-old son was going to play ball with me, and that was that. I plopped him down on the stairs and tossed him the orange moon rock. He ignored me and stared into space. "Catch it, catch it." His hand twitched, a half-hearted move, shudder of a sleeping dog's paw. I moved Ben a few steps down, crossed his legs to make a basket, and set the ball in it. "Throw." He gave the tiniest possible push with the back of his hand. Kerplunk, thud, one step down, ball going nowhere. I retrieved it. "Ben, heads up." It landed beside him. "Throw." He gave me an odd look as if to say, "You want it back already?"

One step forward, two steps back. The forward step is greeted with enthusiasm, cheers, relief. *Now he's getting it, he's on the right track. Attaboy!* The steps back aren't always marked. Didn't he used to say "Daddy" when I came home? Didn't he used to bounce around in his walker like a Hells Angel? Yikes, where *is* his walker? I look around. It's gone.

So it went with the rocking horse, the Slinky, the windup record player: Ben seemed less and less willing to exert even a minimum effort to play with his toys. With energetic prompting—yea, Ben! Let's go, Ben!—he would string a few beads or put a domino through the slot in the plastic top of the coffee can. But he took no joy in it. Unprodded, he'd just sit there. Well, I had a business to build. I decided it best to leave Ben to his own devices, which were fewer and fewer.

He's growing up, we told ourselves. *He's outgrown his exuberant phase; he's more mature, more serious. His interests have changed.* Or, *he's not feeling well today. He has a cold, an ear infection. He's tired. He's recuperating. Give him a day or two.* We had such busy, interesting lives to lead while our son slipped away.

Language, too, was vanishing. Sue and I would prompt him, pointing to objects, naming them, and wait for him to pick up new word. Finally he'd pronounce one, "doggie," as if he'd been preparing to birth it for days and now was delivered of it, perfectly formed. "Yea, Ben! You said 'doggie.' Good for you, Ben." We congratulated each other, relieved. "See, he can talk. He said a new word." Ben looked at us as if he wondered what all the fuss was about and toddled off. So much for *doggie*—that's the last time we heard it. A day or two later out would come another fresh word, "choo-choo," first and last off the assembly line, never to be heard again. Was he going to go through the whole dictionary this way?

One evening I realized that I could keep Ben within my field of vision, fix my eyes on him, but I couldn't *attend* to him for more than a few seconds. *Odd*, I thought. *My kid is invisible.* I tested my theory by paying full attention to Ben and nothing else for a full minute. I held my watch in my right hand and focused my eyes on Ben. He was sitting beside the green woven picnic basket filled with colored golf-ball-size wooden beads: red, yellow, blue. I'd taught him to string those beads, starting with colored pipe cleaners and working up to a thick red and white candy striped shoelace. I'd cheer him on to each bead, each victory. "Yea, Ben!" He'd squeal with pride. But tonight he was not stringing beads. Fifteen seconds into my experiment I realized that my mind had drifted. I was remembering what he used to do. *What is he doing now?*

Nothing. He sat in front of me, staring off into space, his hands dangling from his wrists like tired dog tongues. My attention radar wiped him out, overwrote him as if he were a blot in the blind spot on a piece of paper held eighteen inches in front of the eyes. I tried the experiment again. With determination, I fixed my attention on him for perhaps twenty seconds, then he "disappeared." My son was vanishing before my eyes.

🐚   🐚   🐚

Weekdays, I was under unremitting stress. Balancing baby and business was getting harder and harder. Even on good days, Ben was fussier, more refractory, his eating messier, his colic more persistent, his tantrums more frequent.

Today, I'm at a breaking point. I'm downstairs in the family room at three o'clock in the afternoon, my worst time. My computer is on the floor beside twenty-two-month old Ben, who is watching *The Weather Channel* and keeping an eye on me. Ben is the Motion Police, and I am his prisoner. I am allowed to move my hands a few feet or turn my body within certain parameters, known only to Ben, as long as my butt stays planted. If I stand up, stir, or give any hint that I am about to leave the room, he will start screaming. But I have to pee. Is there a coffee can handy?

Tension had been building all week. On Monday afternoon I'd finished my coffee and walked out the back door, coffee cup in hand. It was part of a set my grandmother had given Sue and me for a wedding present: gray, shallow, with a flat bottom and blue rim around the top and bottom. Deliberately, as if I were delivering the final blow to a nail, I smashed it to bits against the stone terrace. Then I swept up the pieces and hid them in the wastebasket.

Tuesday I wrote "Help" forwards and backwards with lipstick on the mirrors in the bathrooms, downstairs over the bar, and on the white top of the grand piano.

"What's that all about?" asked Sue.

"Nothing," I lied.

On Wednesday, I kicked a hole in the drywall in the hall beside my study. It felt good.

"Dan, what happened to the wall?"

"I kicked a hole in it."

"You're going to fix it, aren't you?"

On Thursday, I sequestered screaming Ben in the bathroom so as not to frighten him. I picked up the hatchet that Sue had been using for a hammer and buried it in the wall like a tomahawk. Frightened—*how could I have done that?*—I fixed the hole with putty and plaster so Sue wouldn't see.

On Friday, I needed to pee. But I'm prisoner of the Motion Police. I plot my trip to the bathroom like a quarterback planning an end run. If I'm lucky, I might be able to get to the toilet and back before Ben rages out of control.

The phone rings, out of reach. Big sale? How can I take the sales call, use the bathroom, and evade another ear-piercing tantrum?

I can't. I cannot do this. I cannot raise this child and build a business.

I muse over this revelation, turn it around in my mind. Surely it cannot be true. *I can do anything I set my mind to, always have. But I cannot do this.*

The telephone continues to ring. Ben is still crying. I go into the bathroom and close the door because I don't want to alarm him. I scream, "I can't do it, I can't do both." I can't. Yet I must.

"I can't," I scream again.

I smash my fist into the bathroom door, breaking through the first layer of fiberboard into the hollow space.

"Christ Almighty."

I kick the wall, the way I had done upstairs, where my foot had made a hole through the Sheetrock. This time I strike a stud. The pain breaks the curse. I limp out of the bathroom. Ben is looking at me as if I have lost my mind, Jack Nicholson over the edge.

I load Ben into the old gray Buick and drive to the north end of Grapevine Lake. I park on a cliff facing the stark winter sunset and watch the water, my toe throbbing, my mind blanked by the pain.

I could just drive in.

DIAGNOSIS

"**H**e's so advanced for a two-year-old!" gushed the teacher.

"Really?" Great. Sue and I had finally found someone who agreed with us.

"In what way?"

"His fine motor skills," the teacher said. "The way he cranks that jack-in-the-box." Ben was still cranking the tinny tune. *Round and round the mulberry bush.* Out popped Jack. Ben squealed.

"He did that all day," she offered.

"Yes, he loves music," I said, shifting the subject.

"I should say he does!" she said. "He could be a composer."

"How about a writer?"

"Or an artist!" Sue chimed in, handing Ben a crayon. "Look: thumb, middle finger, index finger. That's a tripod grip!"

"Hey, Ben. Great first day!" I cheered. "Let's go." *While the going is good.*

"Oh, Mrs. Burns. And Mr. Burns." I should have seen this coming.

"How do you get him to take a nap?"

"We don't," I started to say, stopping myself. *Naps,* I thought. *A big deal at day care, required for tenure.*

"Just burp him and rock him," Sue bluffed. "He'll be fine."

"We tried that but he cried."

And he kept the other kids awake, I thought.

Sue was having no more of this discussion. She hurried us toward the door.

"I'll bring some Gas-X tomorrow. Dan, let's *go.*"

The next day, Ben was in a corner by himself, rocking in his rowboat, staring in the mirror.

"He fusses when we try to make him sit with the other children," the teacher said, glancing at Ben. "When he's crabby like that he crawls to the corner and we just leave him alone."

I didn't blame her. Do Not Disturb a Quiet Baby.

"Did he take a nap?" I asked.

"I've been meaning to talk to you about that, Mr. Burns. No, he did not. Do you have a number where you or your wife can be reached during the day?"

On Friday, at naptime, the teacher phoned me. Ben was screeching like an ambulance siren and the other kids were going off like car alarms.

"He's a lovely little boy," the teacher said. "I'm afraid we can't keep Ben."

I shouldn't have been surprised. I couldn't keep him either.

Sue and I tried Freewill Baptist Academy. The Baptists surrendered by the end of the week. White flag. But Sue and I had no such option. We'd have put Ben in a basket and floated him down the Nile if we thought we could get away with it.

"Dan!" Sue was waving a brochure at me. "I've found a great school for Ben!"

Just what we needed, because he'd been expelled from TLC Child Development Center, where children "experience success on a daily basis," for successfully practicing his Houdini escape act.

"A great new school. Tell me about it."

"It's the Kathy Burke Pre-K Academy for Gifted Learners."

"Yes?"

"It's a drama school. The kids dress up."

I looked at the brochure. Was this a good idea? Gifted. Well, that's Ben: so sensitive and moody, so music-loving, plays his Old King Cole tape over and over, so artistic, decorating the walls with his advanced tripod grip. On the other hand, he didn't play with other children. Wasn't that what drama was all about, play?

Never mind, counseled Sue. According to the brochure, this was an "avant-garde" school where teachers "truly engage the children at their optimum level," where Ben would at last be "appreciated for her or his unique talents and abilities."

Admission by interview and referral only.

Of course, they would never take him.

"Listen, Dan," countered Sue. "It's for underachievers. They take difficult kids."

"What about the naps?"

"Dan, Ben is better. He can take his vibrating mat to school."

"And the referral?"

"Got it." Sue worked for the Park and Recreation Department, City of Dallas. Through her social and professional network she had pulled some strings. We had an interview.

Sue and I prepped him for the meeting. We jimmied the playground gate and snuck into the schoolyard so Ben could get used to the environment, go down the slide, play on the climbing toys. We peeked in the windows, Ben on my shoulders. The school really did seem colorful, new, well equipped.

"This is your new school, Ben. You like your new school?"

If crying was any indication, he did not.

Somehow we bluffed our way through the interview, spinning hope. "Separation anxiety. So sensitive. He'll get over it."

Weekly reports from the school suggested otherwise.

"Ben doesn't relate well to the other children," began the first one. "He wants to be held and rocked."

"Well, hold him and rock him," Sue said through gritted teeth.

One of the teachers, Madelyn, took a special interest in Ben, stood up for him in parent-teacher conferences, pleaded for patience and more time, and gave him the one-on-one attention he needed to get through the day.

The big test for Ben was the Halloween party: lights low, apples in a washtub, spider webs dangling, spooky music, kids dressed for trick or treat. Orange and black masking framed the stage. Imagine Ben's terror. He tried to keep everything the same. He thought the sun should stand still and stop making the shadow of the kitchen table race across the floor.

He made a break for the car, screaming. But we dragged him back into his front-row seat. Waiting to greet him downstage was his good teacher, Madelyn, dressed like a witch. She held out her arms to him, expecting a hug, but Ben shrieked and drew away. Madelyn's face fell. All was lost. It was curtains for Ben.

Next day Sue received a call at work, a summons. One of the staff had observed the encounter with Madelyn and had written it up. *Documentation*, I thought, *not a good sign*. The principal handed Sue a note, more documentation, and told her that Ben wasn't responding age-appropriately. She recommended that we have him tested.

It's a trap, I thought. Kathy Burke was building a case to expel him. The note came with an ultimatum: test him or take him home. The school district had already been notified of Ben's case. It was all arranged.

A few days later I received the news from Sue by phone.

"How did it go?" I asked.

"Ben just cried so they asked me a bunch of questions."

"And?"

"Not good."

That evening I saw the report. It observed that Ben was two years, three months old. In graphic detail it showed that his language, social, and motor skills ranged from nine to eighteen months, with most skills grouped at about a year.

He was testing half his age.

We'd have found a reason to discredit the test—he's right-brained; they test for weaknesses. But the look on Madelyn's face had already told me more than I wanted to know.

❧   ❧   ❧

"Mr. Burns, there's a package for you."

"Oh." I set Ben down under the Eagle Postal Center counter near the jar brimming with cellophane-wrapped red-and-white penny candy. He was waiting for his treat. I removed the cellophane for him.

"Developmentally delayed," the teacher said.

"Developmentally delayed?"

"Significantly."

"Oh."

I see.

The mask was off, the wrapper removed, exposing a child I hardly knew, a snail without a shell. He wasn't cute; he was infantile. He wasn't playing postman; he was trying to escape. He wasn't bright; he was dim as a coal-oil lantern. He wasn't unconventional, charming, or Bohemian. He was feral.

"Mr. Burns?"

He wasn't advanced; he was …

"Mr. Burns, how is your son?"

"Oh, he's … he's …"

Retarded.

Like Donnie, the first-grade dunce who couldn't read the word "breakfast" without saying "breakfast fast." Like Kenny, who came to school with snot on his clothes. I'd heard of families hiding away their mentally challenged members in attics or basements and wondered why. Now I understood.

Shame. Humiliation.

Yesterday Ben was delightful. Today he needed to be rolled back under a log, sheltered from veiled stares, unspoken judgments.

I wanted to get him out, to hide him away from the gaze of strangers.

I'm sorry, Ben. Sorry for the future you may never know you missed. Friendless. Wifeless. Childless. Homeless. I'm just … so … Sorry.

❧   ❧   ❧

It was not his fault, so it must be ours. In the marathon of life, devil take the hindmost, Ben was running at half speed.

Our fault. Through poor genes or a mismanaged, irresponsible pregnancy, we had brought into the world a retarded child.

The good news was that his test scores qualified Ben for enrollment in the Early Childhood Intervention program (ECI) through the Carrollton Independent School District. He could attend the ECI classes at McCoy Elementary, where his sister had gone to school, just a few blocks from where we lived. Ben would be under the care of special education teachers with children like himself, and there would be no more expulsions, because Ben belonged there.

So did we.

Yesterday Sue and I were dressed for success, gussied up, suited and tied, strung with Republican pearls and bound for glory. Today we were in blue jeans and tennies at a parent-teacher meeting at the correctional facility where Ben would serve time.

We were humiliated, incredulous, angry.

To compound our shame, the school offered to send a specialist to our home to show us how to take care of our child.

No, they didn't offer; they insisted. A specialist would visit our disintegrating home. A very young, single, childless specialist, a spy for the school district, would see what a shambles our lives had become.

Kristi Fair, Ben's teacher at McCoy, must have understood our chagrin. She told a story that she shared with every new parent.

"You are on a journey," she began. "You think you bought a ticket to France, but somehow there was a mix-up and your plane lands in Holland. You are shocked, disappointed, angry. You pound your fist. 'I paid for Paris.'"

Yes, that was exactly how I felt.

"But it is a one-way ticket and there are no refunds."

I'm not listening to any more of this story.

"So what do you do?" she continued. "Over time you find that Holland has its own charms: Amsterdam, Rembrandt House. You are glad you found this out-of-the-way destination for its unusual rewards."

Bullshit. I wanted him fixed as soon as possible. That's why we were here, wasn't it?

The in-home specialist gave us good advice. She said, "Make him talk. Don't give him what he wants unless he says the word for it." She showed us how to teach Ben activities hand over hand: "push the train," "turn on the tape player." He was a tactile learner.

How long it would take Ben to catch up? We would just have to step on the accelerator.

≥   ≥   ≥

Most children learn from their peers, especially siblings. By age three, Ben's brother and sister were grown and out of the house—Hannah at Oklahoma State University, Pete married and starting his own family—so Sue and I volunteered to teach three-year-old Sunday school. We could encourage Ben to interact with normal kids his age and learn faster.

It is one thing to fill out a checklist that reveals that your child is lagging in language, interaction, small motor skills, imagination. It is quite another thing to see him side-by-side with normal children. These kids—Kendall, Tanner, Jason, Ashley, Stephanie—were *way* ahead of Ben, little artists and playwrights and architects and musicians soaking up knowledge and learning new skills right before our eyes.

Show Jason how to strum a toy guitar and he thinks he's Elvis Presley. Give Ashley, Kendall, and Stephanie a box of robes and hats, and before you can say "Samson and Delilah" they're improvising dramas. As for the discussions, Tanner said the darndest things.

"If you had been in the Garden of Eden with Adam and Eve, would you have listened to God?" I asked. "Would you have obeyed the rules?"

"No," said Tanner.

"Why?"

Great discussion. Ben wasn't paying attention. When placed in the discussion circle, he crawled away to the corner. When forced to stay, he cried. Now I understood why Ben might want to just hide away in his own world. Who hasn't dreamed of showing up unprepared for the final exam in a course never attended? Every Sunday must have been like that for Ben. In the interactive three-year-old classroom, our son was a non-starter.

Back at home, Sue and I redoubled our efforts to get Ben on the ready-for-kindergarten track. Sue worked with him to identify letters of the alphabet, to match, to point. Hour after hour, day after day, but with no training in behavior modification, no appropriate expectations, no notion of how what she was doing could fit into a larger scheme. She often felt, as did I, that we were on a path leading nowhere. Failure after failure, ear infection after ear infection. We all but gave up.

Sue came home from work exhausted. Made dinner. Vegged out in front of the TV. So did I. We could barely stir ourselves to go to bed.

My nightmare: No matter how hard I ran, carrying Ben, we would never catch up.

🙠　　🙠　　🙠

"We're losing Ben," said his grandmother Dorothy, Sue's mother. It was Thanksgiving 1990. He was a little over three years old.

The realization comes in little shocks, sheet lightning, a thunderstorm still far away on the horizon.

Better keep busy. Grasp at a memory, a fact, a theory that helps you believe for a little longer that what is happening before your eyes is not real.

"I remember when he smiled when Sue and I kissed, how he cooed and cuddled; he's so socially aware."

"His teacher said he was advanced, handled the music box like a kindergarten kid."

"Remember how he worked and worked with the key until he made it fit? And how he laughed when I said, 'Jack jump over the candlestick. Jack Burns!' He has such a highly developed sense of humor. That's the real Ben. He's just going through a stage."

Kristi sent back glowing reports: "I took Ben by the hand & led him to the sandbox. He sat right in the middle of all the children and tolerated all of the noise SO WELL! He had potty accident at 9:30. I bathed him and changed his clothes."

But Ben's attention span was dwindling. He was losing his language. His temper tantrums were increasing. We could not quiet or comfort him. He could no longer feed himself.

Or read his books. Where he used to turn each page carefully— *The Owl and the Pussycat*, *Where the Wild Things Are*, *Goodnight Moon*—now he rifles through them, forward, backward, turns the book upside down, tears out pages.

I explain to the doctors—Ben's Kaiser pediatrician and the specialists he referred us to—and they don't hear me. They offer nothing, not even the cold comfort of the truth. They don't say, "He's regressing; sometimes these children lose their hearing and sight and stop talking; we don't know why. You might as well get used to it because he's headed for an institution and there is nothing that can be done."

No. The lab tests are normal. Neurosonogram, CAT scan, normal. Brain stem hearing test, normal. But this is not Amsterdam. This is someplace I have glimpsed only nightmares, a dungeon in The Hague.

      ❧   ❧   ❧

Most of what I knew about autism was a myth. In the late 1980s I had written and published a scholarly analysis of the rock opera

Tommy, which tells the story of an autistic boy imprisoned in a mirror. Tommy is deaf, dumb, and blind. But he is sensitive to "vibrations," a gift that enables him to become a pinball wizard, then a rock star. With the help of a Dumbledore-like mentor he breaks out of the mirror and is cured.

Sounds like a fairy tale? It is.

Tommy is based on Bruno Bettelheim's psychogenic theory of autism: A child suffers a psychological trauma, withdraws into a shell, and remains there until the spell is broken by a psychotherapist, a modern Dumbledore. The self-imprisoned child is released.

Nonsense.

Bettelheim's theory was tragically flawed. It gave birth to the myth of the "refrigerator mother," too cold and uncaring to raise a functional child. But it made great theater. It also seemed to partially describe Ben: functionally deaf, dumb, blind, in a shell, fascinated with mirrors, and sensitive to vibrations: music, touch, rocking.

Could Ben possibly be autistic?

No, no, surely not.

The very word, "autism," alien-looking and -sounding, struck fear into the pit of my stomach. In the real world, psychotherapy had proved to be 100 percent ineffective against autism. The spell could not be broken. Autistic kids were modern-day lepers, cursed, beyond help, institutionalized for life when they became adults, locked up and forgotten.

I didn't mention the "A" word to anyone. Saying it aloud might subtly alter the quantum structure of the universe and make the worst-case scenario come true.

But the doctors weren't helping, and Ben was getting worse. Someone had to act, research, step into the unknown, descend into the dungeon, rescue Ben.

First we needed to know if Ben was, in fact, autistic. I obtained a checklist from the Autism Research Institute, and Sue and I went down it together.

Looks through people?

"No," said Sue, "but he walks into rooms backwards."

Uses adult's hand to point?

"Yes," Sue answered. "He grabs my wrist and shoves it toward whatever he wants."

Deliberately hits his own head?

"Yes."

Covers ears?

"Stuffs paper wads in them."

Collects odd items? Wire clothes hangers, stems, and knives. *Bizarre pose or posture?* Hangs upside down. *Chews nonfood items, especially metal?*

The list went on.

The problem was that on many points we could answer either yes or no. Sometimes Ben walked on his toes, and sometimes he did not. He avoided interaction with others, but he loved to be held and rocked. Which box to check?

Still ... Running with those coat hangers and screeching. Not making eye contact. Severe tantrums. Sound sensitivity. We'd checked enough *yes* boxes to raise Sue's concern and mine.

As I considered the evidence, however, there were two strong arguments against autism. First, only one kid in thousands was autistic. That meant there was less than one chance in a thousand that Ben was autistic, right? I would bet on those odds any day. Second, if he were autistic, wouldn't the doctors know? In three and a half years, no doctor had even breathed the word "autism."

Wouldn't any competent pediatrician have explored that possibility?

Maybe not. A doctor looks in my son's ears and writes a prescription for Amoxicillin. Another doctor inserts ear tubes and refers us to other doctors, who send us through the labyrinth of the hospital, heart pounding, blood pressure careening, Ben screaming, to take tests.

But no doctor puts the pieces together. No doctor sees the whole child.

And the half dozen doctors we'd consulted to date could not answer even the most basic questions. Why does my son cry so much? Why does he cover his ears with his hands? Why does he tear up books when he used to love books? Why does he whisper when he talks, and why did he stop whispering?

🐚　　🐚　　🐚

I shared my concerns about autism with Ben's Kaiser pediatrician, who referred us to Dr. Nancy Hitzfelder. She was one of the few pediatric neurologists in Dallas who saw autistic children. It was December 7, 1990, my birthday. Ben was three years and four months old.

If we had a diagnosis, I felt, we could fix Ben.

"Autism, a tough case!" I imagined Dr. Hitzfelder saying. "We've got to reverse the downward spiral."

"How?"

"We'll take a three-pronged approach," she'd say, scribbling on her prescription pad. "Genetic, neurological, metabolic."

"Great."

She'd rip the sheet off her pad. "Here," she'd say, handing it to me. "Call Children's Hospital and schedule a glutathione infusion. I'll alert my colleagues and arrange a complete workup." She'd pick up the phone. "We'll get to the bottom of this!"

"What about speech therapy?" I'd ask.

She would finish punching numbers into the phone and look up at me. "Ben may not need it," she'd say cheerfully. "Many of these children start talking after the first push."

That is not what happened.

Dr. Hitzfelder picked up a blue beach ball and set it in front of Ben.

"Kick the ball," she commanded.

Ben did nothing.

"Kick!" she repeated.

Ben seemed not to hear.

Dr. Hitzfelder turned to me. "When did you first notice that Ben was developmentally delayed?"

"Developmentally delayed" was too clinical a term for the nightmare that had brought us here. For the first year and a half, I explained, Ben was eccentric but more like a normal child, though fussier, messier, and more exuberant than his older brother and sister. By eighteen months, pencil in hand, he had covered the walls of his room with fancy lines and intricate loops. He was going to be an artist for sure, or maybe a writer. But at about twenty months his tripod grip had twisted into a fist, and his loops had shriveled into scrawls. Then he stopped scrawling.

And talking.

Now, on his better days, Ben would spend hours waving a pencil in front of his face or looking in the mirror and making motorcycle noises.

"Does he resist change?" the doctor asked. She was making notes.

"Yes, he doesn't even like me to move."

I explained that Ben was the Motion Police, and I was his prisoner.

"I see," said Dr. Hitzfelder. She made another note. "Is he getting any assistance through the school system?"

"Yes, some."

Kristi was grasping at straws. "He stopped masturbating and got out from under the easel when I told him to," her last note said. "He didn't verbalize any words for us but he did make eye contact for a second when I said his name."

We were losing Ben.

Dr. Hitzfelder stopped writing.

"Well?" I asked.

The doctor hesitated, weighing her words. "Ben does demonstrate a number of clinical features of autism," she said carefully.

"Does that mean he's autistic?"

"Too early to say." She was warming to her subject. " It is difficult to separate autism from mental retardation, especially for a severely impaired child like Ben. In either case, it is doubtful that he will ever achieve normal developmental potential."

"What is the treatment?"

"There is no medical treatment for autism or mental retardation."

"No treatment?" I repeated. "That's it?"

Dr. Hitzfelder sighed wearily. "Some parents are experimenting with diets and other non-medical interventions," she said. "I'll give you contact information for the Dallas Autism Society should you decide to follow that route."

How could diet and "non-medical interventions" cure a brain disorder? I wanted teams of doctors, ambulance sirens, surgery, drugs.

One more question. "What about speech therapy?"

Dr. Hitzfelder leaned forward, as if to speak confidentially. "I have seen many parents like you spend a small fortune on speech therapy for children like Ben." She leaned closer.

"My advice to you is to take him home, love him, and let the school system look after him for as long as possible. Save your money for his institutionalization when he turns twenty-one."

PART 2

THE JOURNEY

SUNRISE

The collision with Dr. Hitzfelder whiplashed us into action. There had to be a medical treatment for Ben. She had just not been keeping up. Sue and I were going to beat this thing.

"Dan, the doctor didn't say he was autistic."

She didn't have to.

I supposed Dr. Hitzfelder was trying to spare us. For her, the word *autism* was a label that would lock Ben forever in a padded cell, no medical treatment, beyond help. For me, it was the key that would let him out.

The battle began.

Sue and I had a secret weapon. In the early days of the Internet, few doctors had network access. But I had a dial-up modem.

Screech! Bawk! I logged into Medline, gateway to five thousand biomedical journals, and typed in "autism." A stream of green letters scrolled across the screen: "Clonidine, an Alpha-adrenoceptor Agonist, Reduces Melatonin Levels in Mice."

Hieroglyphics. Would Clonidine help Ben? The article didn't say. How about the next article? Hundreds of titles. Which of these arcane texts contained clues to the cure? I was going to need a medical degree to decipher the mind-numbing jargon.

As the floor piled high with dot-matrix printouts, hour after hour, it seemed that Dr. Hitzfelder had been right. The research journals gave us little snippets of knowledge that didn't add up. One hundred and fifty pieces of a thousand-piece jigsaw puzzle, a worm's- eye view. But nobody, it seemed, was looking at the big picture. Had any of these researchers actually seen an autistic child?

Sue and I were just going to have to plow through the articles, put the pieces together, look at the big picture, and come up with a cure. But like nearly everybody else in the 1990s, we thought that autism was primarily a brain injury caused by a genetic defect. We knew that in addition to Ben's weird behaviors and lack of speech, he had colic, hypersensitive hearing, allergies, sleep disturbances, and chronic ear infections, but we didn't necessarily see those symptoms as part of the same picture.

The Ultimate Stranger, the book I'd found in the Carrollton Public Library, was the closest thing we had to a big-picture theory of autism. "He is an alien in our midst," Delacato wrote of the autistic child. "He almost seems possessed by some nonhuman power that compels him to carry out his own alien acts of self-destruction."

Yep, I thought, *that's my son.*

Could it be, asked Delacato, that these repetitive behaviors, these "autisms," carry a hidden message? That these children are not psychologically damaged, but brain injured, like some institutionalized children who are blind or deaf?

Brain injured? Could be.

Could these *stims*, short for self-stimulatory behavior, be the child's attempts to reestablish sensory intake channels for sound, sight, taste, smell, and feel?

Yes. Yes. Yes, it could be. Yes. That's it!

Ben bit his hand, screamed, slapped his face, and ate his own feces because he was attempting to treat himself.

And the treatment? Sensory integration: systematically stimulating the senses. "As the sensory channels are normalized, the strange repetitive behavior ceases," wrote Delacato.

Made sense to Sue and me. I wondered what other parents of autistic children thought about it.

I went to a meeting of the Dallas Autism Society. Someone read the minutes—incomprehensible, full of alphabet soup, MHMR and AZT and PR1026—to an auditorium full of other parents seeking relief. During a break I approached one of the well-dressed speakers.

"Excuse me," I said. "Perhaps I have come to the wrong place." I had his attention. "People here seem to be talking about obtaining support services for their autistic children," I went on. "I do not want support services for my autistic child. I do not want an autistic child. Where is the room for people looking for a cure?"

"Oh, you must be new. I'd like you to meet my son, Thomas. He's relatively high functioning. Say hello, Thomas."

"Guhg," said Thomas. He sounded like a pig barking.

I'd stumbled into Purgatory.

"You'll get used to it," said the father.

No, I will not get used to it, I thought. How can I listen to these lectures on the politics of advocacy, the probable funding level for Texas State Bill 1594, the inclusivity debate when I am trying to save my son?

"I've seen these fads come and go," the father continued. "Every few months it's some new cure. Right, Thomas?"

"Guhg."

"I have an appointment with Dr. Delacato in Pennsylvania," I said. "What do you think of his Sensory Integration Therapy?"

I could see that the father was about to warn me off, but he didn't want to discourage a newbie in the autism society and changed his mind.

"Why don't you go to your appointment and let me know what *you* think."

That was all the encouragement I needed. On April 17, 1991, Ben and I hopped an American Airlines flight to Philadelphia.

Delacato had retired from clinical practice, but he recommended that we meet with his colleague John Unruh, Ph.D., who would evaluate Ben and design an individualized rehabilitation plan.

At first sight, the Centre for Neurological Rehabilitation car-alarmed my puff detector. Its grandiose name, the European spelling of "Centre," and its clip-art logo of a satellite circling the Earth suggested a high-tech international venue. But the center was housed in a modest low-rise office building in Morton, a working-class town outside Philadelphia. The letterhead listed half a dozen doctors as consultants, including Delacato. But the working staff seemed to consist only of John Unruh and a clerk named Mrs. Unruh.

If the Unruhs were surfing a publicity wave generated by *The Ultimate Stranger*, it had long since washed back into the ocean. Ben and I were the only visitors in the clinic.

Well, nothing wrong with a family business. Or with a Ph.D. But doubts nagged. Was this a Potemkin village? Where were the CAT scanners, the galvanometers, the strobe lights, the AudioTron? "We have software right here in this clinic that doesn't exist anywhere else in the world," bragged Dr. Unruh.

Who doesn't? I thought to myself.

If the Unruhs could actually help Ben, I'd gag my doubts and stuff them in an incinerator.

Dr. Unruh reviewed Ben's medical history while Ben played around the old wooden desk. On it were Ben's folder, a pair of earmuffs, and a yardstick. Dr. Unruh stood up, put on the earmuffs, picked up the yardstick, and hid it behind his back. When Ben wasn't looking, Dr. Unruh slapped it soundly on the desk.

Bam! Ben didn't flinch.

"Aha," said Dr. Unruh. "Auditory dysfunction!"

Ben scooted under the desk and peed on the carpet. End of evaluation.

Dr. Unruh's "individualized rehabilitation plan" consisted of a mimeographed sheet of instructions pulled out of a file drawer. The promised "orientation" was a discussion of how to implement them. Ben and I had come a thousand miles for this? I was disappointed.

But at least we had an agenda, a place to start.

Back home, Sue and I squeezed Styrofoam panels into the window, hung a swing from the ceiling, and padded the floor with wrestling mats. Ben's room became our sensory integration lab, his funhouse.

We formed a tag team so we could keep him busy every second. The goal was to keep his attention focused outside himself.

We followed Dr. Unruh's instructions exactly. We whispered in Ben's ears, rolled him up and down the mats like a log, swung him, spun him in a swivel chair, tucked his head under his shoulders and rolled him in somersaults. We ran our fingers over his face, rubbed him with a dry towel, tipped his tongue with lemon juice, sugar, and salt, hoping to open the sensory channels.

Lights off, room dark as charcoal, we crossed the air with the colored penlights. Oh, and deep pressure. Sue and I knelt by his sides. We squeezed his limbs, all four of them, our fingers and palms tightening like blood pressure cuffs. "Deep," Dr. Unruh had counseled, "but no pain." Twice a day. For a month.

Ben loved the exercises, especially the log roll and limb squeeze. He'd laugh gleefully, and we'd get a little bit of eye contact. At least the therapy gave Sue and me a structured way to relate to Ben.

Did it reduce his "autisms"? Without a baseline and a data-tracking system, it was difficult to tell. Maybe his attention span really *was* a little longer. Feces smearing and masturbating continued unabated. Big effort, small result.

Dr. Unruh sent a letter to remind me that we were supposed to meet with him four times a year for re-evaluations and changes in the treatment plan. At best, he counseled, sensory integration was going to be a "long-term program" that "does not offer quick results."

What must we do to get quick results?

❧   ❧   ❧

"Dan, look at Betty Lou's letter," Sue called to me from the next room. "Here's a story about an autistic kid who got well."

"What?" I was impatient. Ben's great-aunt was always sending us news articles, clippings, more stuff to toss on top of piles of reading and research materials we accumulated on our own.

"It's called *The Sound of a Miracle*."

Great, another miracle. But this one could not be ignored because it had been published in *Reader's Digest*. The author, Annabel Stehli, told how her autistic daughter, who had hyperacute hearing, was "freed from autism" by listening to distorted music.

Why not just go to a witch doctor.

"It's all in the sensory processing part of the brain," Stehli explained. Hyperacute hearing is a sensory dysfunction. As for AIT, Auditory Integration Training, it was a tough sell, the author admitted. "Like trying to pitch AA in a barroom."

Stehli's daughter was reportedly cured in ten hours.

Interesting.

The article led me, via the Internet, to the Institute for Child Behavior Research, a low-profile information clearinghouse where Stehli worked. The institute hadn't shown up on my radar screen because it didn't have "autism" as part of its name, and the older search engines just weren't powerful enough it pick it up. The institute's director, Bernard Rimland, had a Ph.D. in psychology and an autistic son. He had written *Infantile Autism: The Syndrome and Its Implications for a Neural Theory of Behavior*, which demolished Bettelheim's theory of the "refrigerator mother" and launched the search for biomedical treatments. Operating on a shoestring, Dr. Rimland had made it his life's mission to discover useful therapies by putting parents of autistic children and research scientists together.

Somehow Dr. Rimland had acquired my address and had sent me a handwritten note offering an advance copy of a book, *Nobody Nowhere*, and some papers on autism. I knew nothing about the man or his work. But that was about to change. I ordered back issues of his *Autism Research Review International (ARRI)*, a kind of *Reader's Digest* for parents of autistic kids. Dr. Rimland and his editors combed through mountains of medical journals and summarized discoveries that parents and clinicians could use. They clarified the jargon without dumbing down the content, sniffed out trends in research and explained their importance, highlighted political and educational developments, and put them in perspective. *ARRI* included lists of papers and information packets that parents might find useful, each for just a dollar or two to cover postage.

Over time, Sue and I came to trust *ARRI*, each issue a gift of hope; but at first it was just another resource, one voice among many. If vitamin B6 plus magnesium was good for autism, and if twenty-six scientific studies supported that conclusion, as Dr. Rimland claimed, why hadn't Dr. Hitzfelder mentioned it? Why was there "no medical treatment for autism," and why hadn't the B6 studies popped up on our Medline search?

We started Ben, age three years and ten months, on a low dose of vitamin B6. We also started a daily 125-milligram tablet of DMG, dimethylglycine, a vitamin-like food that, according to Dr. Rimland's parent surveys, jump-started language in about 40 percent of autistic kids. But these were just vitamins and nutrients. Having witnessed the life-changing power of pharmaceuticals—penicillin, the Salk polio vaccine—we'd keep hoping and searching for another wonder drug, a silver bullet, a cure.

Dr. Rimland sent me another handwritten note—didn't the man own a typewriter?—inviting me to try various therapies Sue and I were researching on Medline and to share my observations with him. Yes, I would gladly collaborate. I would experiment on Ben, safely of course, and inform the good doctor which therapies were working and which were not.

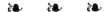

"Dan, here's one."

Sue was working the computer, Medline, and had pulled up "Antidepressant and Circadian Phase-Shifting Effects of Light: Correlation of Family History with Specific Autistic Subgroups." Autism had been shown to occur more frequently in families with bipolar disorder and seasonal affective disorder (SAD). My mom had both. Could autism and SAD be different manifestations of the same underlying disease? We'd noticed that Ben got better in the summer as the days lengthened and worse in the fall as they shortened.

Exposure to artificial sunlight—phototherapy—helped some patients with Seasonal Affective Disorder, and we'd tried it on Mom. Perhaps, as he neared his fourth birthday, it would help Ben, too.

It was a straw, and we grasped it.

At least phototherapy was something we could *do.*

Sue got Ben up at five o'clock, set him in his high chair in front of the video player, and flooded him with a Vita-Lite. As the sun rose I'd take him on a baby jog to the park, racing his stroller over the roughest parts of the sidewalk to the edge of the wood-planked bridge. I'd pause to let Ben anticipate the bridge, back up for the launch—he'd gasp—then one, two, three, *race* across as loud and fast as we could go, *clatter clatter clatter clatter wheeee,* and back over the arched planks toward the rising sun. After breakfast under the Vita-Lite we continued remnants of the sensory integration therapy: swinging, chair whirling, deep pressure. We also raised his DMG to 250 milligrams a day.

Ben rallied.

Some of his language resurfaced: *uh-oh, doggie, mama.* He talked to his cousin Morgan on the phone, saying "me me me me me." When his brother Pete came to practice with his rock band, Ben jumped into his arms.

"Hi, bro!" said Pete. He twirled him and tossed him, as usual, always glad to see his baby brother, but this time Ben was trying to talk. "Ah ah, boo, too ..."

We hadn't heard babbling like this for years.

Encouraged, we added 500 milligrams of vitamin B6 plus magnesium to Ben's daily regime. It was difficult to get him to swallow the foul concoction. Sue mixed it with ketchup and put it on his eggs or moistened Cheetos and dipped them in the B6 powder. We managed to get at least half the recommended dosage down him—sometimes.

Progress continued. Ben stopped crumbling his sandwiches. He matched items on his Touch & Tell, and he experimented with a Nintendo. He played bite-my-hand with a monkey puppet. He threw Popsicle wrappers in the trash and played the piano with his toes. When Ben saw Sue get the big dinner pot out of the oven, he said "Hooray!" Lying in bed between us at night, when he should have been sleeping, he whispered "baby, baby, baby."

Week after week the surprises just kept coming.

Early in July, I noticed Ben watching me mow the lawn. When I walked away from the mower to pick up the garden hose, Ben took over. He grabbed the lawnmower handles and pushed. Is this my son? I could scarcely believe it. Last time I mowed the lawn he ran away from the clangorous contraption.

At the library, Ben sat still and played with a dinosaur puzzle. A week earlier he'd have pulled down books, screeching. Today, he was calm. And something else seemed to be different about him, something physical, the way he looked and moved.

"Ben, bring me the book."

Ben stood up and walked toward me. Yes, that was it: his gait. Instead of walking on his toes, or stomping and swaggering, he lifted his leg and put his foot down on the heel.

"Ben, let's go outside."

There, on the library lawn, he looked taller, straighter, surer. I pulled a ball out of the back seat of the car and rolled it across the lawn. "Ben, get the ball." He ran toward it like a normal little boy.

Late in July, Ben produced a torrent of words. During his shower that Thursday morning he said, "Hey." That had become his way of asking for attention.

"What?" Sue answered.

"Bye-bye big boy," said Ben, meaning he wanted to go to his Big Boy School. "Dan, drive him to school!"

You bet!

That evening, at the dinner table, Sue asked him, "You ready for your dinner?"

"Yes," said Ben, "ready."

Sue put a steaming plate of spaghetti in front of him.

"Hot!" said Ben.

"I'll cool it off for you," Sue answered. She blew on the spaghetti and handed him the plate. "Try it now," she said.

"Hot," Ben argued. "Hot, hot."

"You want me to blow on it again?"

"Yes," said Ben.

"Ok, I'll blow on it. See? Is it all right now?"

"Yes. All right!"

It was his longest conversation since he'd stopped talking. Today, a month before his fourth birthday, Ben was again using words to communicate. Ben was recovering not only language, but small motor skills, social skills. No wonder his summer-school teacher was sticking the *attaboys* on his folder.

Hope was returning to our lives. Sue and I finished the picket fence we had been building. I sent a letter to Dr. Rimland describing Ben's progress and detailing our work with phototherapy. Oh, and the vitamin B6.

By the end of July, Sue and I had decided to make potty training our number one behavioral goal. "Ben's lack of potty manners," I wrote in my diary, "is holding him back. In daycare, he cannot be promoted out of the diaper room, and the older kids make fun of him. Potty training might put an end to his feces eating, one of his least endearing traits." I set a one-year goal: "By the time he's five, no more diapers."

I put aside my distaste for Skinner's boxes and ordered Dr. Rimland's articles on operant conditioning, also known in autistic circles as Lovaas therapy. According to Dr. Rimland, operant conditioning was practically foolproof. You, the teacher, break the target skill into small steps and reward successively accurate approximations of each step, coupled with occasional use of "aversives," such as a loud "No!" Operant conditioning, he said, works on cats with half a brain and works on slugs if you are patient enough. Autistic kids, too. Once a few behaviors have been taught the child begins to learn on his own. He has learned how to learn.

Sue and I teamed up on Ben. I specialized in poop training. I made careful note of Ben's bowel movement times and taped a roll of Sweet Tarts over the toilet. When he was ready to go, I'd rush him to the bathroom, install him on the pot, and wait for him to finish his business. Then I'd pop him a Sweet Tart.

Sue specialized in pee training. She'd give him a drink and sit him on the pot every twenty or thirty minutes until he had finished his business, then Sweet Tart him.

Within a few days Ben was using the bathroom by himself and pulling up his pants. Once when I forgot to give him his Sweet Tart, he snatched the roll of candies off the wall and gorged himself. That was his graduation present. I'd budgeted a year but Ben was essentially potty trained in about a week.

The McCoy fall semester was starting in two weeks, just after Ben's fourth birthday. Kristi had warned us that children in the Early Learning Program don't catch up with their peers; they just fall behind more slowly. At this rate, Ben was going to hop the train. He was good to go.

I began to enjoy my time with Ben. I mounted a child seat over the rear fender of my bike and in the evenings, at dusk, Ben and I took off. From our garage door behind the house the driveway sloped steeply, launching the night ride as we picked up speed; then the decline gentled out and Ben and I would coast all the way to the park, sometimes steering to port or starboard through the maze of streets and alleys in our new subdivision, which a year before had been field of cattle and mesquite. As the bike picked up speed, Ben squeezed my arms and squealed his high-pitched, delighted "Wheeee!" We sailed to the west, hair whipping, toward the rising moon. I was a pilot, but this was more fun than flying. "The *moon!* The *moon!*" I would enthusiastically proclaim, echoing *The Owl and the Pussycat*. "They danced by the light of the *moon!*"

We were no longer prisoners. We were Elliott and E.T. flying through the night sky, free.

SUNSET

But even as Ben rallied, the stress on the family was taking a toll. July of 1991, Sue and I entered family counseling, trying to save our twenty-four-year marriage. As summer blended into fall, our relationship continued to unravel.

July 23, 1991. Sue and I met with Russ Dunckley, Ph.D., a family therapist, to discuss some issues in our relationship. Sue and I had struggled repeatedly with my sexual orientation, beginning before we were married. She knew I was gay—my affair with Joel was no secret—but marriage was supposed to keep me on the straight and narrow. An unlikely expectation, from a twenty-first century perspective, but one that we held on to in spite of all evidence to the contrary.

By late summer of 1991, I was losing control. Beneath the fortress of our marriage, tectonic plates were shifting. I dreamed about a small city in Iowa, like Iowa City, where Sue and I had lived during our first three years together. In my dream, a building collapsed, burying hundreds. Then the top half of a glass-and-steel tower imploded. Workers down by the river were drilling a deep hole for a pier, and the limestone substrata carried the force from the drilling in to the city. In the dream, I watched slow-motion films of one building falling. On the top floor, the walls cracked open, and I could see the people being pummeled by debris as the walls and floor gave way.

In real life, Dr. Dunckley was drilling into the substrata of our marriage. On August 2, 1991, he talked to Sue about her having come from an abusive background, and when he asked if she had been sexually abused she become very angry. She was unable to recall sexual abuse, but the question was very upsetting for her.

August 18, 1991. "Hold up four fingers, Ben. That's right, you're four years old!" On Ben's birthday he was coming down with a cold.

August 19, 1991. On his day-after-birthday, Ben received his four-year immunizations. He was sick. The doctor noted that Ben had "no eye contact," was "known to have autism," and was "scream-ing all the time." Nevertheless, Ben received three vaccines: for oral polio; diphtheria, tetanus, and pertussis; and measles, mumps, and rubella. One month later, at the request of the school, Ben received his Haemophilus b conjugate vaccine.

August 25, 1991. Ben began the regular fall semester of his Early Childhood Intervention program at McCoy. "He reentered the Early Learning Program," I wrote in a letter to a friend, "and met all of his first year developmental goals immediately. His teachers are as-tounded. So are we."

August 30, 1991. Our marriage counseling continued. Sue re-called some sexual involvement with her father as a child and said she was angry with all men. I supposed that included me.

September 6, 1991. Which therapy was helping Ben? I said vita-mins; Sue said light. Careful to keep our disagreement from spilling over to Ben, I wrote to Dr. Rimland for advice. He suggested that we try one therapy at a time and observe the results. We took Ben off B6 and DMG. "By the third week in September," I wrote in my diary,

"Ben was 100% un-potty trained and was using no language except 'eee-Up!' He was masturbating like mad." All systems were failing: potty training, language, attention span.

Could removing vitamin B6 and DMG have caused Ben's regression? That seemed like an obvious conclusion to me, but Sue was heavily invested in the phototherapy. She took pride of ownership in her web Medline discoveries because she put two and two together and had come up with a novel treatment. Through our online network we were sharing our observations with the parents of other autistic children and with several doctors, including Dr. Rimland. It was exciting to think that we might be medical pioneers on the forefront of discovery. So Sue and I ramped up the phototherapy, substituting artificial sunlight for the waning autumn sun. Sue worked with Kristi to set up phototherapy for Ben at school. I bought a light meter. We kept data.

November 5, 1991. I wrote, "Attempts to replicate last summer's light therapy results have not been successful …We charted Ben's behavior in potty training, masturbation, commands, eye contact, socialization, and use of language. After more than two weeks, there was no clear improvement in his behavior on the light therapy compared to baseline behavior in the categories we charted." Ben had cratered. We put him back on vitamin B6 and DMG.

It's tempting to assume that Ben's four-year vaccinations were at least partially responsible for his regression. Mercury, which was used as a preservative in Ben's vaccines, is a potent neurotoxin, and some children may be hypersensitive to its damaging effects. In addition, the measles, mumps, and rubella shot has been said by some researchers to leave a chronic infection, "gut measles," in the digestive system of vulnerable autistic kids. If so, in this scenario, the infection puts the immune system on permanent alert and floods the blood with antibodies, bombers on a misguided mission, engines flaring, attacking and inflaming the brain. But in 1991, vaccines were not suspected as a trigger for autism. Because Ben's regression didn't occur immediately after the shots, Sue and I didn't suspect a link. All we knew was that we were at the bottom of the crater, and Ben wasn't responding to the B6 and DMG either. We were stuck.

Thanksgiving 1991. Our marriage counseling entered a critical phase. As I wrote in my diary, "I am not giving Ben the time, attention, or empathy that I was for a while in July. Sue and I are busy working on our marriage."

"Struggling with our marriage" would have been more accurate. Occasional infidelities had become hazardous. I had already given Sue a herpes infection. HIV was epidemic in the gay community. What if I gave Sue AIDS? That would be tragic, unforgivable. Longer term, and more surely, my little trysts were taking a toll on me. When I look at photos from that era, my mom's favorites, I scarcely recognized myself. Who had I become? A liar and a cheat. The fortress of our marriage had become a prison. Sue and I discussed it. The only solution we could see was to break out.

New Year's Eve 1991. Sue and I were upstairs in the master bedroom, Sue's pantyhose streaming from the ceiling fan. It was near midnight. We were drinking André champagne and listening to live jazz from the Caravan of Dreams.

"Dance, dance, dance," urged Sue.

I was self-conscious, sad, couldn't get into the mood. Nothing fit, nothing seemed right. Another fault line had shifted.

"Just dance and you'll feel like dancing," Sue insisted.

I went into the closet, closed the door, then opened it again and limboed my way out.

"If you're coming out of the closet," she said, "I'm leaving."

The next day, Sue bought me a present: two brandy snifters. "For you and your next boyfriend," she said, "to toast."

January 4, 1992. That Saturday, Sue made good on her threat. She packed her personal belongings in a U-Haul and drove away.

Though the failure of the marriage was largely my fault, I was not prepared for the cataclysm that followed. The morning Sue left it seemed like the end of the world. I lay down on the guest bed and the sound came swooping out of me as if from someplace deep inside … Nooooooo-o-o-o … like wind sweeping out of a cavern, Carlsbad Caverns, the flight of the bats at sunset swirling out of the bowl-shaped mouth of the cave, my mouth, then rising in a whirling funnel, endlessly rising as if being sucked from a bottomless pit, the cave's very entrails. NooooOOO-o-o-o … My marriage. My family. My son. My hopes and dreams. Sundered. NooooOOO-o-o-o … And Ben, the child that I'd wished for upon a star, was left to free-fall into the abyss.

⤳   ⤳   ⤳

Sue rented an apartment near her work and we took turns taking care of Ben, three nights on, three nights off. That arrangement gave us some much-needed relief from Ben's constant demands and his control as Motion Police.

From my office at home, Mondays through Wednesdays I'd volley software-marketing proposals out the door, backhand the mailbox, buggy-whip the phone lines, and cannonball the Internet. Thursdays, though, Ben and I pile in the car and drive, well, anywhere to get away from the turbulence I'd created. We'd explore off-road villages, one-shop towns, paint-peeling backwoods burgs in northern Texas or southern Oklahoma, detritus of the postwar boom, looking I suppose for Mayberry, for Brigadoon. We found Jefferson, Texas, petrified in the 1860s, but our favorite destination was Turner Falls, a place that had changed little since my childhood: Honey Creek, the great basin at the foot of the falls, steep and deep, the rock-ribbed ancient mountains, the cedar valleys, the circling hawks. Ben loved brooks, flowing water, fountains, rain, pools. We'd climb the flint trails and look down at the falls from across the valley. I found in this sacred ancient vault a rootedness, a peace of mind, a sense of being that would, I thought, outlast us. When my brief candle flickered out, I thought, the hawks would circle still.

Back home, marketing *Thoughtline*, my speechwriting software product, I surfed on waves of cash flow. High tide, when the money rolled in, I flew from coast to coast participating in trade shows and television interviews, a gambler on a binge. I'd predict sales that were off the chart and imagine a warehouse full of *Thoughtline* packages, shipped by air around the world. Low tide, when the money rolled out, I wrote speeches for Texas Instruments (TI) executives and produced annual reports for Dallas oil companies. I paid down debt and waited for the surf to rise.

Boom and bust cycles in Dallas were the norm, and I fit right in. When the economy turned up, I'd late-pay the mortgage so I could buy postage for thousands of sales letters. Same with the car. I'd skip a payment and plead with Ford Motor Credit for one more chance. Out went the letters and back came the orders, my mailbox stuffed with checks, enough to pay the debt and them some. Risk? In my view, an economic recession was just a dry spell between cash flow surges. I hung on to the dream that a wave of sales would carry me over the top, the million-dollar mark, and I'd sell the business.

It was a relief to get Ben out of the house half time and to shed the suit of armor, my heterosexual persona, which had become so restrictive, a burden. Sue was enjoying her freedom, too.

"You both act like you've just been let out of prison," Mom observed.

But what was the effect on Ben? I had learned from potty training Ben that he needed a consistent set of rules to shape his behavior. I was a drill sergeant. "Close the door," I'd say. "Pull up your pants. Flush the toilet. Turn off the TV. Put on your shoes." But Sue was a laissez-faire mom. She allowed him to use his hands even on the messiest food: scrambled eggs, rice, macaroni and cheese. Occasionally, Ben, Sue, and I would eat out together.

"Ben, use your fork," I'd prompt.

"Dan, let him be!" Sue would argue. Her point was that it was better to let Ben eat with his hands than not eat at all.

I had learned from raising my older children that unless parents agreed on the rules there were, in effect, no rules. How would Ben react when he moved from the laissez-faire environment of Sue's apartment to my house, and back?

March 1992. Three months after Sue split, I'm monitoring four-and-a-half-year-old Ben as he eats his breakfast cereal with a spoon, which he is perfectly capable of doing as long as he is watched. Closely watched. Superdog barks; I shift my attention to the door, then back to Ben, the flick of an eyeball. His hand flashes into the milky bowl of Rice Krispies, which are dribbling out the ends of his fist. His stealth radar detector alerted him when my attention strayed.

Using the same extraordinary stealth powers and sleight of hand, Ben learned to open doors and vanish. A moment's inattention and he'd break out running in a straight line, heedless of his caregivers, never looking back. If not collared he would cross all barriers— creeks, fences, fallen trees—like a guided missile honing in on a target. Perhaps there was some unheard music, some Pied Piper, some siren song attracting him. From inside our house Ben could vanish like a garter snake, slither out an unlocked door, slip through cracks and crevices like a cockroach. He's upstairs decorating the walls, right? No, our neighbor is on the phone, calling me because Ben is foraging in her refrigerator. On a walk around the block he'd jump out of his stroller and run like a Dallas Cowboy toward some stranger's front door, me dashing after him to make the tackle.

Just to see how far he would go, I watched Ben cross an open field. He tromped through mud and climbed over a barbed wire fence toward the woods until I, afraid of losing sight of him, zoomed off and made the arrest, a motorcycle cop chasing a speeder. Ben had covered a good city block. Where did he think he was going? Was he looking for his mother? No, he ran away from her, too.

Ben lived hand to mouth: he taste-tested everything he picked up, then tossed it wherever he happened to be. He sniffed out pasta with the enthusiasm of a dope addict looking for a fix. I tied a lasso around the fridge; when that failed, I bolted a padlock to the door.

Ben's shirt, during the brief time it was on him, was covered with the remnants of meals. He seemed to have at least three hands, all of them dirty, and he wiped them on the walls and in his hair.

When Ben became bored with a toy, he would toss it over his shoulder or pitch it down the stairs. Breakable items were tested for durability by breaking them. He dug through closets and scrambled under beds looking for clothes hangers and sticks to add to his collection. Ben preferred to run around the house naked. Drawers were for pillaging, cabinets for plundering, clothes for shedding. He tried to flush the cat down the toilet.

As Ben's activity escalated, I became hypervigilant. I'd lunge for the glass before it fell, secure the door before he ran out of it, grab the ketchup bottle before he dumped it on his food, lock the gate, hide the bread, bury the jelly jar under the dish towels. In my haste I'd spill the milk and splatter the ketchup.

In response to Ben's escalating misbehavior, his Kaiser pediatrician referred us to a psychiatrist. "I can write you a prescription for Ritalin," she said. Sue and I had heard that Ritalin was a chemical straitjacket. We put aside our reservations. We'd have accepted a physical straitjacket if she'd offered it. But Ritalin didn't work. It made Ben more hyperactive.

How to work at home and keep an eye on Ben? I ripsawed his door in half and left the top open, turning his room into a horse stall. He spent the days corralled there, trying to remove the window screen, smearing feces on himself, the walls, and the carpet, rending his books, and sticking spit wads in his nose and ears. He'd regurgitate his food, chew it like cud, and spew it out.

How could one kid cause so much destruction? Days off, I'd clean up the wreckage. I made a note to rip out the carpet and power-spray the walls.

Mom came to visit on Ben's fifth birthday and we surveyed the destruction of my home. No longer a prisoner, I had my freedom, but at a terrible price. From unfathomed falls of grief, this poem came tumbling out.

To Ben on his Fifth Birthday
August 18, 1992

Your room, once hopefully prepared, in disarray,
Your chest with missing drawers like broken teeth,
Expelling clothes too large, so small.
Blue handprints jellied on the wall.
Your favorite blanket sprawled upon the floor,
Twisted like a chromosome astray.

These things matter to you not at all, nestled fast
In your waking dream still among the reeds.
Time's river flows right past.
You're five. Your childhood will not stay or last,
Ebbing just as, word by word, your language slips away.

Do you, like Wordsworth, live in wonder,
Yours still the constant hour
Of splendor in the grass, of glory in the flower?
And do you yet long for that celestial bower
From whence you came? I tour the house,
Remembering your favorite things:

To eat a grape, your Wee Sing tape,
Your swing, a clutch of pennies scattered on the floor,
The telephone, Rice Krispies, a scarlet flower,
Your playful bite, the moon at night,
Air brushing past your ear as you cycle
On the seat held tight.

Outside, by the broken swing, a blue jay scolds
The neighbor's cat in our unweeded yard,
Once carefully rolled.
Your trike lies where it fell among the grass,
A tilted gravestone. When you rang the bell
Last night you spent your final word, moon.
A sign? Are you going home so soon?

Oh, do not leave the playful light,
Your perfect body, brown and bright.
Oh, do not leave the broken room,
The slighted yard, the cycling moon,
Your cradle in the reeds at night.

I walk the terrace. Seen from above,
Ants trace a trail of Krispy rice.
Tears flow. Can this be love?
Remembering, I see the moon
Reflected in your wondering eyes.
Can this be Moses, Christ?

Ben completed the summer session at Jose Navarro Elementary School, a temporary assignment, and was to be reassigned for the fall term. He was five years, three months old. His teacher, respected for her work with autistic kids, was about to be interviewed on KERA-TV, the public television channel for North Texas, but she took the time to go over Ben's report card with me. "Remains seated at group table: unsatisfactory. Parallel play with peers: unsatisfactory. Eye contact: zero. Attention span: he doesn't have one." She set down the list and stared straight at me.

"In twenty-five years of teaching Special Ed," she said, "Ben is the most autistic child I have ever seen."

Though we were separated, divorce pending, Sue and I worked together on Ben. At the school's request we had him tested again. On October 27, 1992, Sue called me to give me the results.

"Well?" I prompted.

"They said he is severely autistic."

"Yes?"

"And profoundly retarded."

It was the lowest possible rating: not just a failing grade, a mere F, but a zero, untestable.

"They offered him a special classroom at Walnut Hill Elementary," Sue went on. "It's a Total Communications Unit."

"What's that?"

"It's something for kids like Ben," said Sue.

Yes, I thought. It's where the school system puts kids they've given up on. A warehouse for untrainables. A room with no windows where the door stays closed.

Dr. Hitzfelder's parting words came back to me. "Save your money for his institutionalization," she had said. "He'll never function beyond a four-year-old level." We'd spent three years trying to prove her wrong, but she was right.

It took some time for the news to sink in. At low tide for my business, I was supposed to be writing speeches for the chairman of

TI. I took my coffee and yellow legal pad to the courtyard, where I could look like I was working, and wept.

"You're grieving," my therapist explained. "The child you thought was yours has died. You must get on with the grieving process. You must work through your grief to get past it."'

❧   ❧   ❧

Ben's window looked out to the west, over the labyrinth of alleys below where we used to ride our bikes, toward the rising moon. Late in October 1992, Ben tumbled out the window, fell a good ten or twelve feet, and narrowly missed the sharp stones we had used to extend the patio and the pointed ends of the picket fence on the other. Using up two or three of his nine lives, he landed in the soft flower bed, stunned and angry but otherwise uninjured. He was dangerously out of control.

Sue and I took Ben to see Dr. Debra Hockett, the psychiatrist who had put him on Haldol, Anafranil, and other medications to try to control his hyperactivity. "It's not working," I told the doctor. "We think he needs to be hospitalized."

Ben made the case for us. Dr. Hockett's office became his amusement park, the couch his Tumble Bug, the office chair his Tilt-A-Whirl, the window his House of Mirrors. He bounced from wall to wall like a racquetball. He dove over the couch into a pile of yellow legal pads and tore out pages. He mounted the desk, tried to climb the mini-blinds, and nearly succeeded in pulling them down. "Sit!" I ordered. I pulled him away from the window.

"Let's stabilize him," said Dr. Hockett. Sue and I enthusiastically agreed.

On November 3, 1992, five-year-old Ben was admitted to Timberlawn, a psychiatric hospital for children, for a twenty-eight-day stay. He was given a Clonidine patch. I was relieved because I knew that Ben was safe. I could take care of my business without fear that the next car horn I heard was going to be followed by a splat.

When Sue and I went to visit him, a few days later, I expected to see him in a straitjacket. But he was clean, calm, and collected. A staffer told him, "Go to your room," and he complied immediately. Once inside he waited at the threshold, as if facing an invisible door, toes just inside the mark.

"Hi Ben," said Sue. "Mommy brought you a present. You want your present, Ben?"

Ben wanted his present, but he wouldn't step over the sill. He was waiting for the staff to give him permission to come out.

Over the twenty-eight days, Ben's behavior improved. He was discharged with a Clonidine patch. Sue saw that patch as a badge of hope, something tangible that we could take with us. But I had suspected that it wasn't really the patch that had transformed Ben so much as the orderly environment, the consistent set of rules. Unfortunately, we couldn't take that home.

⁚   ⁚   ⁚

By the winter of 1992, the business tide was rising again and cash for *Thoughtline* was flowing in. Looking at the sales projections, I thought, why not just double everything? Send twice as many letters. Make them twice as long. Print them in red. In the early spring of 1993, I borrowed against house, car, and credit cards, sent out 30,000 letters, and waited for the checks to roll in. Back came two or three orders, next to nothing. It was a wipeout.

"Trust thyself," wrote Emerson in "Self-Reliance." "Every heart vibrates to that iron string." I'd hitched my wagon to a star, imagined myself as master of my fate and captain of my soul. I had believed that if all of Dallas perished in the aftermath of a nuclear holocaust, I would somehow find a back road to Lost Creek Bluff and live there self-sufficiently with my family, as I once had lived in the backwoods of Canada. I'd believed that if the whole fury and might of the enemy—autism—were arrayed against me, I like Churchill would fight on the beaches, in the fields, streets, and hills, and that I would never surrender.

But now the time for surrender had come. In March 1993, Ford Motor Credit had called and said, "Leave the key in the front seat and the window down. We'll come by to pick up the car." In April, the sheriff had tacked an eviction notice on my door.

On May 15, 1993, the long-pending divorce was final. By August, my business, or what was left of it, belonged to the bankruptcy court. My son was a lunatic, wild as a cheetah, and dumb as a stone.

On October 25, the final blow: Dad died. I listened to Bach's *Mass in B Minor*, Mozart's magnificent *Great C Minor Mass*, and Andrew Lloyd Webber's haunted, grief-scarred *Requiem*. I became the booming drum, the heartbeat echoing in the hall of grief. Dad used to say, "When I want to know the cause of my problems I just look in the mirror." Now I understood. My life was a train wreck, and every piece of debris could be traced to a decision I had made.

Where did it end? The iron string, "Trust thyself," had snapped. Having made so many bad decisions, how could I expect to make good ones? I was paralyzed with fear. If I stepped on a crack, would it break my mother's back? Which parking spot might bring me bad luck, or good? Which words spoken or unspoken might careen me into a fresh indignity, the final loss: Ben?

That would be unbearable.

If I couldn't trust myself, whom could I trust?

"Abba," I prayed, "open my heart, open my mind, open my life." The prayer was both a plea and a confession. "Abba," as my church, the Cathedral of Hope, taught, was the intimate word that Jesus used for a heavenly parent, Daddy/Mama. "Open my heart" acknowledged that I closed myself off from everyone in grief, need, want, and pain, even myself. "Open my mind" confessed that I needed a radically new way of thinking. "Open my life" was an admission that the boundaries I had set to protect myself had become a prison. I took a job teaching writing at Eastfield Community College. And I prayed as I had never prayed before.

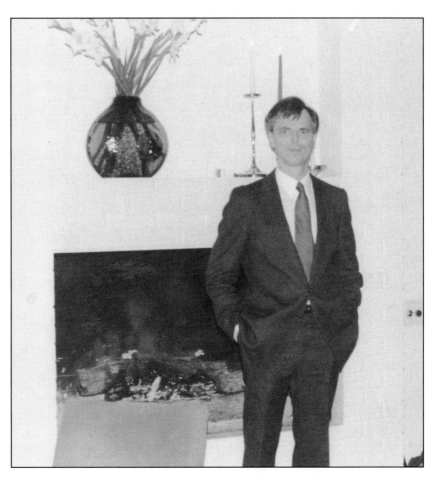

Dan Burns, before the storm.

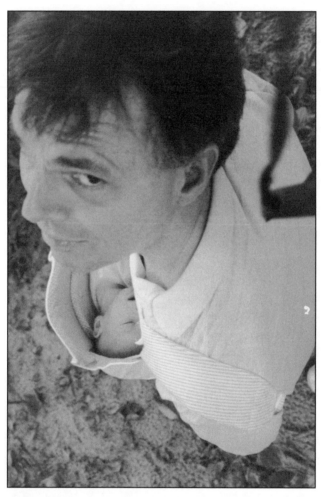

Ben lay at the bottom of the baby bag, a kangaroo pouch, his head size above the 99th percentile.

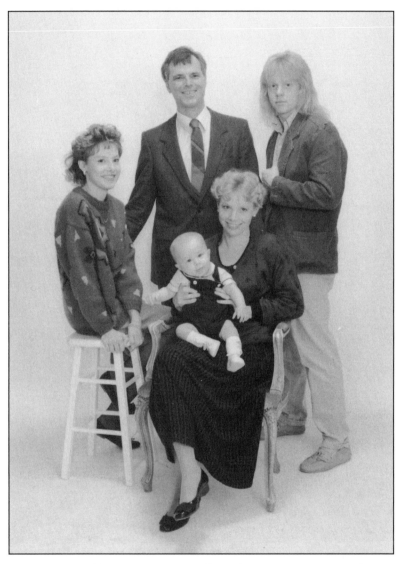

Family portrait: *(clockwise, l to r)* Hannah, Dad, Pete, Sue, Ben. Sue and I were dressed for success, a trope on *Ozzie and Harriet*.

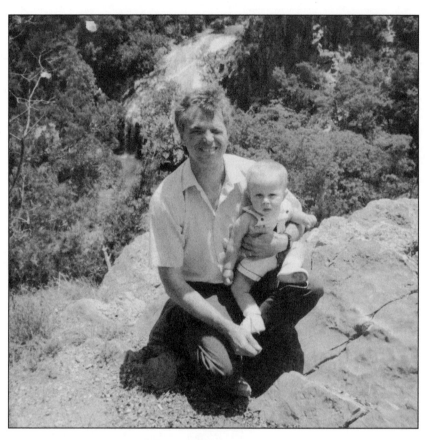

First annual trip to Turner Falls in Oklahoma.

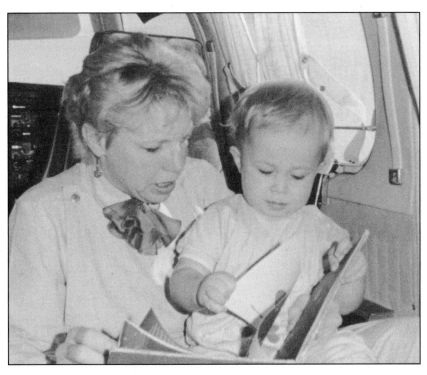

Sue and Ben read *Goodnight Moon* in Grandpa Richard's airplane.

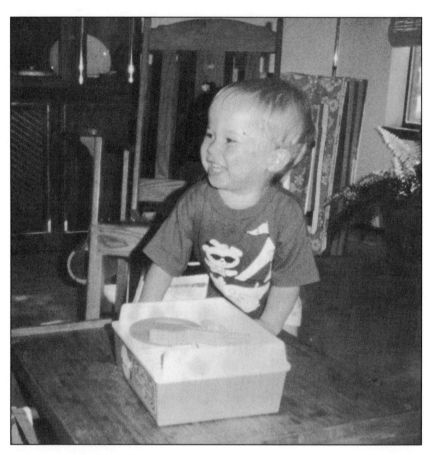

Ben and record player. He loves music.

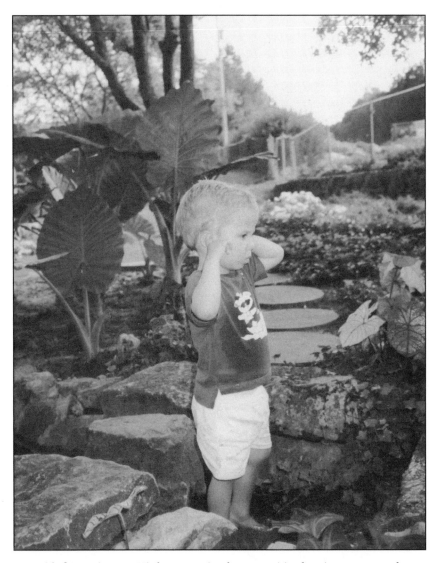

Ben with fingers in ears. His hyperacusis—hypersensitive hearing—worsened at about age one.

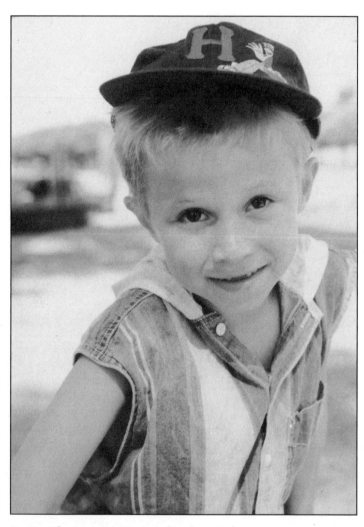

Starting The Benjamin Project: "Look at Me."

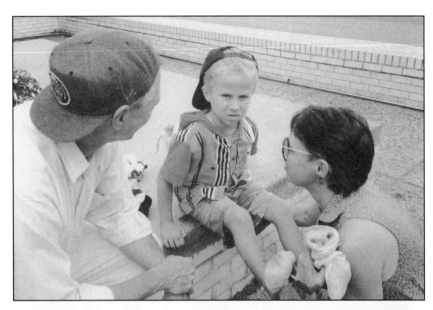

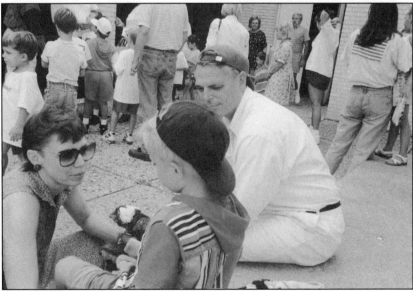

Ben, Sue, and Dad outdoors, two looks.

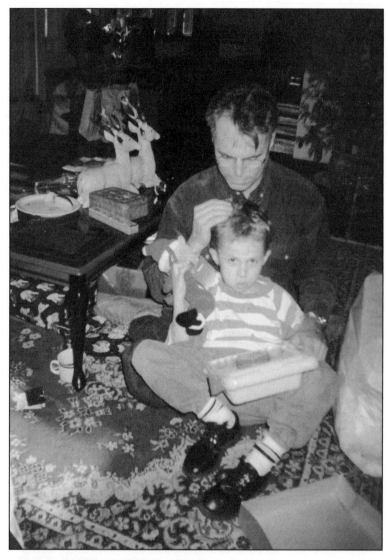

Christmas at Dorothy and Mary's house.

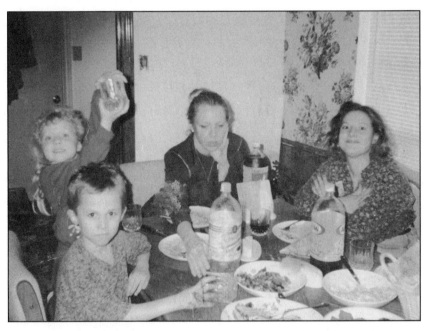

A family dinner. Ben spilled his drink. *(Clockwise, starting front left)* Ben, his niece Morgan, Sue, and his sister Hannah.

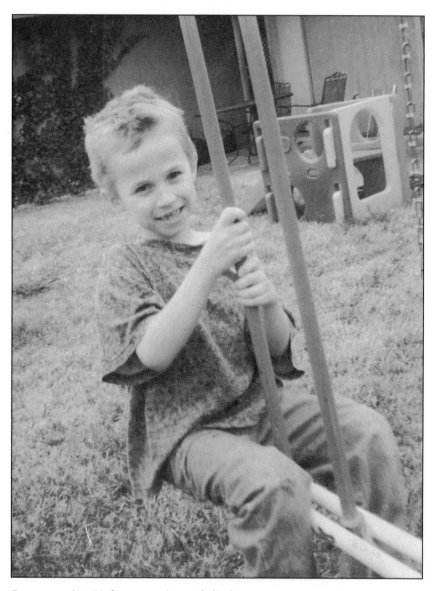

Ben on a swing. He loves to swing and climb.

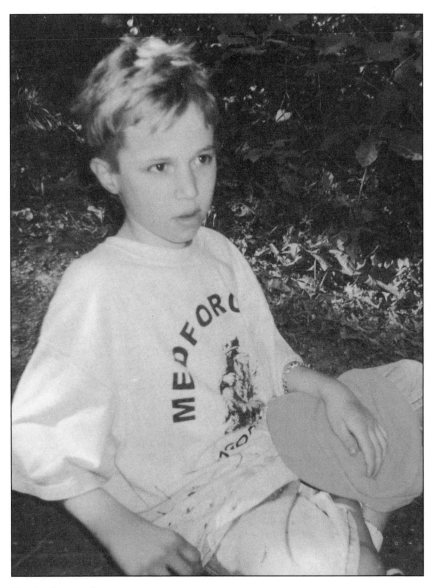

Ben in the woods.

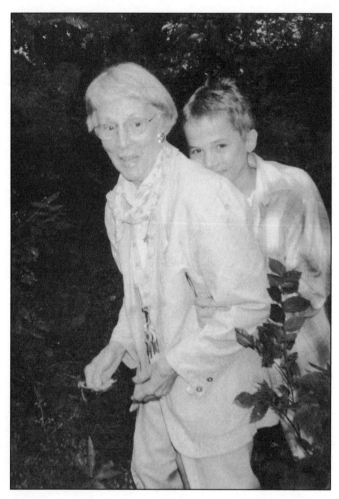

Ben plays hide-and-seek with Grandma Jeanne.

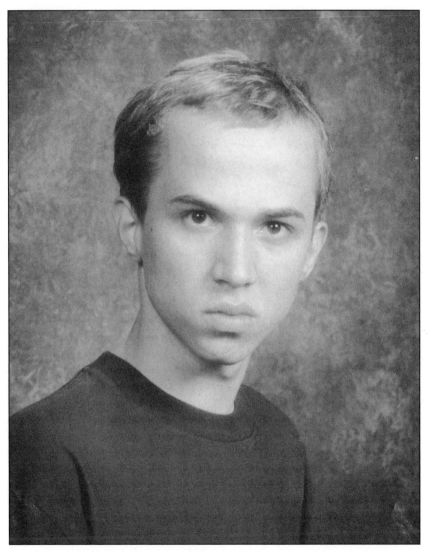

Ben's annual Sears portrait at age fifteen.

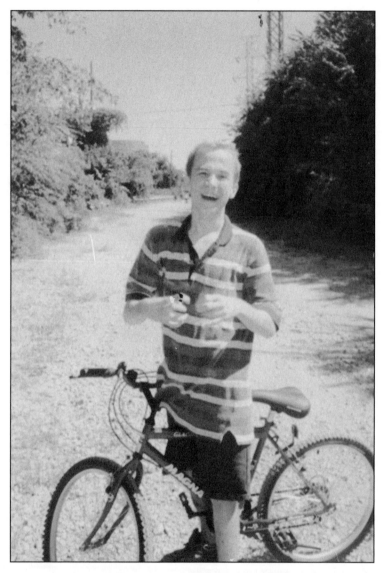

Ben bikes the Katy Trail with his dad three or four times each week.

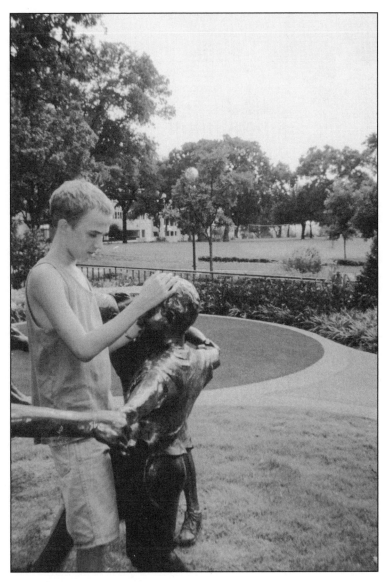

Ben loves children—here, with a sculpture of a child.

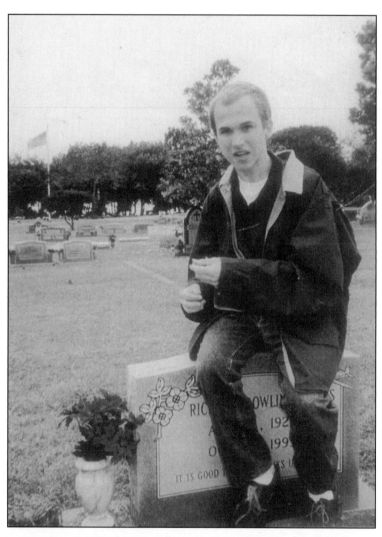

Ben on Grandpa Richard's gravestone.

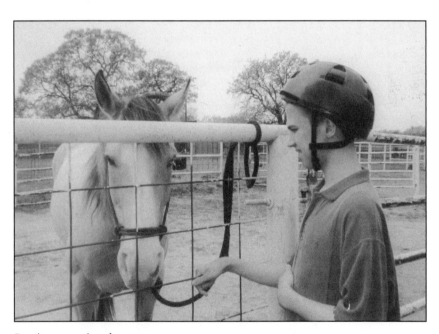

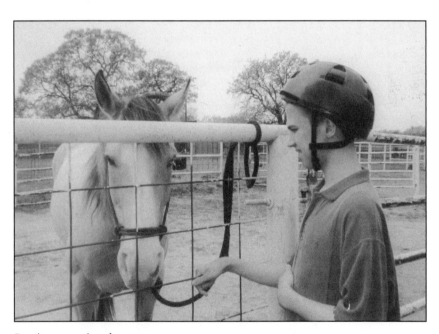

Ben in equestrian therapy.

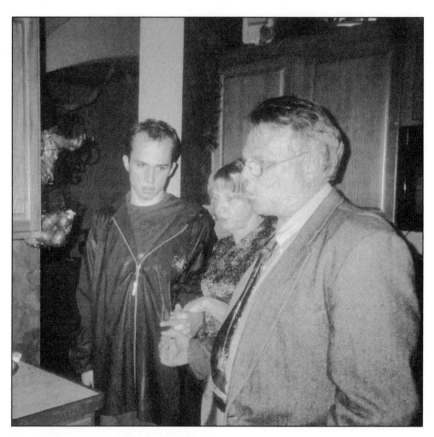

Ben, Sue, and Dan during the holidays.

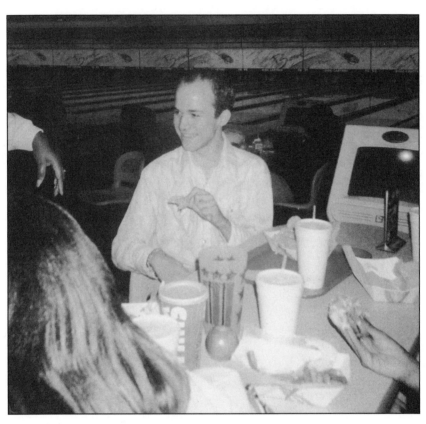

Ben enjoys bowling and snacking with his teachers.

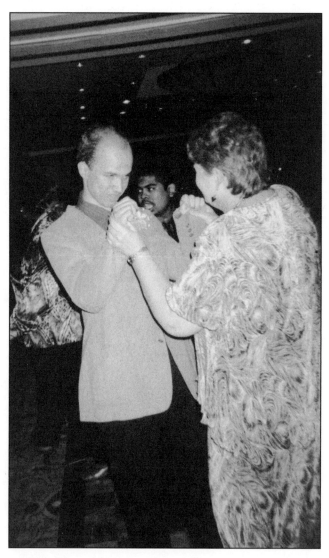

Ben dancing at school prom, age twenty.

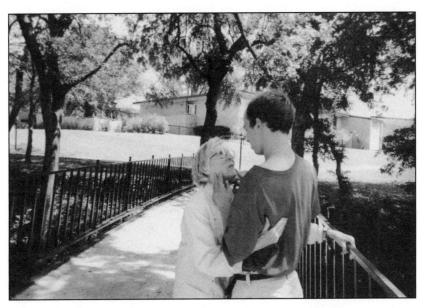

Ben says goodbye to Grandma Jeanne at Grace Presbyterian Village.

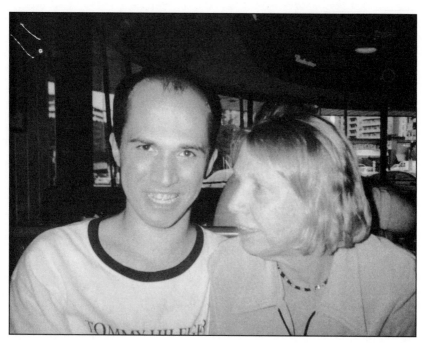

Ben and his mom at Lucky's Café.

PART 3

OZ

SIT, QUIET HANDS, LOOK AT ME

July 1993. I pulled into the parking lot of Walnut Hill Elementary School, the Total Communication Unit where five-year-eleven-month-old Ben was housed. His new teacher, Ms. Seevers, had called me. She was waiting for me in the office. I was not looking forward to meeting her.

"Come with me," said Ms. Seevers. "I want you to see something."

What trail of destruction had Ben left behind him now? As we walked to the portable building, the cellblock, I apologized for Ben's behavior. "He's off his medication. It's making him worse. We've tried everything to control him."

Ms. Seevers swung open the door and there was Ben, standing on the seat of his little desk chair, waving a drumstick, and screeching like a power saw.

"Sit," the teacher commanded. Ben sat down. She took the drumstick away from him and gave him a piece of goldfish cracker. He waved his hands in front of his face and hummed like a band saw. "Quiet hands," she said. He rested his hands in his lap and stopped humming. "Look at me," said Ms. Seevers. To my astonishment, he *did*

65

look up at her expectantly. "Good job!" she said, smiling and holding his attention with her eyes. She gave him another piece of cracker.

I wouldn't have been any more astounded to see Helen Keller spelling out "water" at the pump.

"How did you do it?"

"Discrete trial teaching," said the miracle worker. "You break the behavior you are trying to teach into small parts and reward each part."

"Then you put the parts together." I said. "Lovaas therapy."

"Yes!"

"That's how I potty trained Ben!"

"He's potty trained?"

"He used to be. When he was three."

"You ought to take a look at the UCLA videos, Mr. Burns. Dr. Lovaas is recovering autistic children."

I ordered the Lovaas videos from UCLA but couldn't wait for the mail. Posing as a medical student, my pocket weighted with dimes for the copy machine, I crept into the University of Texas Southwestern Medical School library and made my way through the labyrinth of shelves until I found the *Journal of Consulting and Clinical Psychology*. I pulled the volume from 1987, the year Ben was born. On page three was the article I had been looking for: O. Ivar Lovaas's "Behavioral Treatment and Normal Educational and Intellectual Functioning in Young Autistic Children."

Wrapped in the gauze of passionless academic prose was a revolutionary message: "47% of the experimental group [those who had received the behavioral therapy] achieved normal intellectual and educational functioning … The recovered children show no permanent intellectual or behavioral deficits and their language appears normal." They were mainstreamed into first grade. They became, in a phrase that was to echo throughout the autism community, "socially and intellectually indistinguishable from their peers."

Lovaas therapy did not involve diet, surgery, or drugs. How could behavior therapy—essentially drills—heal a ravaged brain?

Were the children misdiagnosed? Did Lovaas make a mistake? Some clinicians thought so, but over the next decade, the study was to be been replicated time and time again. Consistently, almost half the treated kids recover. Most of the others benefit significantly.

A discovery that cures autistic kids! Why hadn't Dr. Hitzfelder mentioned this article? Or Dr. Rimland? Why weren't Ben's doctors e-mailing me copies? Why weren't school administrators holding seminars and handing out packets to Special Ed teachers?

Soon enough, I would see firsthand how the medical and educational professions, especially autism specialists, deal with prophets who challenge their creed. "Autistic children do not recover," they believe. "All else is nonsense." Because if they do recover, the piers on which these doctors and educators have built their careers would sink in the sand.

But in the summer of 1993, it was Ben who was sinking.

❧   ❧   ❧

"Fasten your seat belt," I command. Five-year-old Ben fumbles with it. "Fasten it, like this." I push the lock together; it snaps shut. "You do it." I unbuckle the belt and put the ends in his hands. "Fasten," I say. More fumbling, then nothing. "Push."

"Ahhhh."

"No, hard. Push hard, like this." I grab his hands and push the lock together. "Do it."

"Ahhhh."

"Do it!"

"Ahhhhgh!"

I am boiling with frustration. I turn away from him and pound my fist on the roof of the car, hard enough to hurt. I know he can buckle his seat belt because I'd seen him insert the clip into the slot. What he cannot do, or will not do, is push it hard enough to snap the lock into place.

Ben cannot operate a tape cassette player because he can't, or won't, push the play button hard enough to make it engage. He can't, or won't, slam a car door with enough force to close it, nor can he pop open a soft-drink can. Why? He'd had screwdriver fingers as a toddler, and a grip like a bear trap. But by age five, if the gumball machine knob didn't turn on the first try, if the gate didn't smack shut or the TV channel selector didn't crank to the next number with a minimum effort, carefully rationed, Ben excused himself; the task required too much commitment, too much risk, too much investment of himself in the real world. Why bother? He quit trying.

So his responsibilities shrank. We had taken over his feeding, his toileting, even his play. Where did it end? As I stood in the driveway it was clear to me: Ben could drift down the river of life all the way to a state institution, where no one would ever bother him again.

Or I could fight for him.

"Fasten it."

Ahahahahhahhhuuugh! Ben is crying in astonishment. His eyes widen and his sweet face begs, *No, no, I can't do this, please don't make me do this.* In his eyes I have become an utter stranger; no, worse, something transmogrified, a werewolf, because what I have been doing is a betrayal of an unspoken contract: that I will shield him from frustration as well as from harm. Breaking the contract, I have turned into a monster. But at this moment I don't care. I will do what it takes to get my son to fasten his seat belt, because I know he can do it, and because all hope hangs on the outcome.

"Buckle it."

"Ahuuuugh!" Ben claws at himself. He bites his hand until the blood comes, and he bangs his head with his fists. His own cries choke him; he cannot get his breath.

"Jesus God," I whisper. It is a curse and prayer, and with it I enter another realm of being, one in which I am infinitely patient, as serene as a stone saint. I gulp air. I squat down at eye level with him. "Ben, fasten the belt," I say with a madman's smile. "Fasten it, fasten it, fasten it." I repeat the phrase in exactly the same tone of voice, infinitely patient and forbearing. I prepare to repeat it all day. "Fasten it. Fasten it." Ben cannot hear me because he is screaming.

I sneak a look around. If anyone witnessed this scene I would be dragged to the loony bin. But we are alone, and I am as methodical and implacable as a stoplight. "Fasten it."

"Ahhhha."

"Fasten the belt."

"AHAHAAHAH." He is screaming at the top of his voice now, poking the hook at the slot, jerking his hands back and forth, missing half the time, but pushing harder. "Fasten it."

"Ahahahaha."

"Fasten it. Fasten it."

Now he is red with anger, his face covered with snot and tears. Defiant, enraged, he thrusts the hook into the slot with all his strength. It buckles with a satisfying *clack*. Surprised, Ben looks up at me. His face shows astonishment and pride. Thank you, Ben. Thank you, Jesus God. We won.

🐝   🐝   🐝

"What's this?" I asked. Sue had come to drop off Ben.

"It's a book Martha gave me," she answered. *Let Me Hear Your Voice,* by Catherine Maurice, with a foreword by Bernard Rimland. It had been buried under junk in the back seat of Sue's car for the past few weeks. I read the subtitle: *A Family's Triumph Over Autism.*

I went up to my study, turned to chapter one and read straight through the next 244 pages. Maurice told how she and her therapists, using Lovaas's forty-hour-a-week intensive therapy model, had dragged her afflicted children kicking and screaming from the Ninth Circle of Hell. A mother warrior, Maurice quoted Donne:

> Batter my heart, three person'd God; for, you
> As yet but knocke, breathe, shine, and seeke to mend;
> That I may rise, and stand, o'erthrow mee, and bend
> Your force, to breake, blowe, burn and make me new.

For Maurice, autism was a battleground, just as I had experienced in the driveway with Ben. She'd expected nothing but blood, sweat, tears, and the possibility—just the possibility—of full recovery. And she got it.

I closed the book at three o'clock the next morning.

If Maurice did it, so could I.

🐚   🐚   🐚

I took down Ben's ceiling swing and cleared the room until it was bare as a boxing ring. In the center were Ben's desk chair and my beanbag chair. I surrounded the beanbag with training materials: watch, yellow legal pad, pen. I was armed with Lovaas's *Teaching Developmentally Disabled Children*, popularly known by its subtitle, *The Me Book*, which Maurice had used to recover her children. And a coffee saucer of green grapes cut in halves.

In his chair sat Ben, howling. I kneeled in front of him. "Arms up," I commanded.

He did nothing.

I grabbed his hands with my fingers and raised his arms. "Good!" I said as if it were all his idea. I stuffed half a grape into his mouth. "Good arms up!" He paused to swallow, then resumed howling.

Again I commanded, "Arms up!" This time I grabbed only his fingers and used the minimum lift I needed to raise his arms. "Good, Ben. Good arms up!"

Grape, gulp.

I repeated this routine five times, touching his hands more and more lightly each time, fading the physical prompt until at last I was not really touching him all. Still, his arms went up on command. I took data, four hash marks and a cross. Five out of five, ten out of ten, twenty out of twenty.

Ben had learned. Soon enough, the howling ceased. He was enjoying the game.

And so was I. As a potter shapes the spinning clay smoothly and surely to the arch, so I shaped Ben's responses. I taught him "touch nose," "touch ears," "pat head." For six minutes, I'd lock onto Ben.

My sight, hearing, touch were tuned to him as if we were a single organism. I had not only a sense of power but also a sense of the exact limits of power, its boundaries. Like building a tower of blocks, intricately balanced, I pushed to the edge of the possible, then stopped. I had to feel my way, know when the blocks were about to tumble. I sensed when to draw back, creep or plunge ahead, take a break, review, consolidate, celebrate. I was connected to Ben like a compass, dancing to the magnet of his moods.

"Pat head, Ben. Good patting head!"

Grape.

When the six-minute burst was over I fell back into my beanbag chair, spent, a machine gun nest surrounded by the data I had been taking. Though Ben initially resisted, threw a tantrum, his resistance was futile. I thought of Dr. Rimland's observation: "A slug can learn if you are patient enough." Learning was occurring on a neurological level far deeper than Ben's untempered will. I was reaching deep into the organism, beneath his disorganized behavior, down to the cellular level, down to the level of individual neurons, rewiring him as surely as if I were using a soldering gun.

There is a scene in *Star Wars* where Luke Skywalker prepares to fire a missile into the port of the Death Star. He locks his sights upon it. Nothing exists for him but the target, because the Force is with him. So it was with me. I was no longer helpless against autism. *The Me Book,* which detailed the therapies behind the story told in *Let Me Hear Your Voice,* showed how to teach behaviors from "raise arms all the way" to language and complex social skills. Nothing could stop me. I had patience, tools, power. I could teach. Ben could learn.

The Force was with me.

With power came an increased sense of urgency. In theory, there was no limit to what Ben could learn, but there was a practical limit. The children in the Lovaas experiment had been ages three and four. Lovaas had targeted preschool children so the recovered ones could be mainstreamed beginning with the first grade, before the school system imposed its own inflexible demands. Ben was six, which was still, by some imaginative stretch, preschool age. He would be seven in four months. Beyond that, first grade could not be postponed. Could Lovaas's results be stretched to include a child age five? And if so, could they be stretched to age six? Age seven?

Years had been lost. I felt that Ben was slipping in over the sill of language just before the window was slammed shut. If mainstreaming him into first grade were the goal, every day counted. How many teaching opportunities, how many discrete trials, could I cram into sixteen waking hours in the next four months? I knew that I couldn't do it alone. Even if I had been able to walk Ben single-handedly through the entire Lovaas curriculum, his new behavior would have to be retaught, generalized in each environment. I was going to need all the help I could get. And that presented problems.

In his foreword to *Let Me Hear Your Voice*, Dr. Rimland had warned that some professionals and parents believe that "the mere imposition of demands and structures on a handicapped child equates to abuse." How true. All Ben's life we had made allowances for him. We helped him with little tasks by completing them for him, like setting a glass of water on the table without spilling it. We allowed him to dash off from the refrigerator where he had been foraging without closing the door, to run back and forth across a room unchallenged, coat hanger in front of him, screaming like a kamikaze pilot. We had been patient with him when he tore the pages out of books. We refrained from pressuring him to pick up objects he had dropped. Because of his disability, we conceded him the right to grab food off others' plates.

In the new, recovery-is-possible world of behavior modification, I understood, like a blind man who has at last received his sight, that all of these defeating habits had to be broken. Not just Ben's habits, but also our family's. I met with fierce resistance every step of the way.

I drove Ben to his mother's apartment carrying Ben's little chair and green grapes in a bowl. Sue met me on the patio.

"Look," I said, "Ben can learn!" I showed her his growing repertoire: sit, look at me, clap hands, raise arms, touch nose. She was impressed.

"How did you do it?"

"I'll show you." I positioned Ben in front of his little chair. "Ben, sit," I commanded. He did. I knelt down in front of him. "Stomp feet," I ordered. As I expected, Ben did nothing. I grabbed his ankles and stomped his feet for him. "Good stomping feet, Ben," I said, and gave him half a grape.

Sue went inside her apartment and closed the door. "I can't watch this," she shouted through the window.

"Why?"

"It reminds me of being abused."

Undeterred, I drove to Ben's grandmother's house. In the comfort of her living room, I taught Ben a simple imitation: stand up. He sobbed as I had expected and eventually stood on his own, no physical prompt. He had learned. Still sobbing, he reached out for his little reward, half a grape. He knew he had earned it.

I was elated. Mom was horrified. "The poor child. You're harassing him. Don't push him. Let him be!"

I explained to her that we had let him be for six years, and he was getting worse. So what if he protested, resisted, howled. Do you want a placid child or a recovered child, I asked. He'll get over the sobbing. My son who was given up for lost is back.

That night my aunt Betty Lou called me from Florida. "Jeanne is distraught. What did you do to Ben?"

When Betty Lou hung up, my brother, Cris, called. Instructed by his church to shun me for being gay, he made an exception in this case. Mom was beside herself, he said. She was calling everyone in the family, telling them I'd gone mad. I was torturing Ben.

"You're doing the right thing," said Cris. "You've got to get down in his face. But you must never, never drill Benjamin in front of Mom again, or even discuss the drills with her."

I was in this alone.

Although I hadn't used it yet with Ben, there was a component of the Lovaas program that frightened some parents and educators: the use of mild aversives such as a shouted No! to suppress tantrums. As the parent of most any autistic child will tell you, a tantrum is a seismic event that can be measured on the Richter scale. Its nickname, "meltdown," suggests Three Mile Island, Chernobyl, the implosion of a nuclear core, "an emotional outburst," as *Wikipedia* puts it, "wherein the higher brain functions are unable to stop the emotional expression of the lower brain functions … an irrational fit of crying, screaming, defiance, and a resistance to every attempt at pacification in which even physical control is lost." The child turns inside out. The rebellious reptile brain shoots the czar and his family and—raging for revenge— lets loose the dogs of war. When that happens, Lovaas suggests using an aversive to suppress the tantrum long enough to redirect the child.

I learned the value of aversives by experience. Ben decided to throw a fit in the library. I know from experience that he is capable of sustaining a tantrum for hours.

But I am ready.

Ben collapses on his butt, screaming and biting his hand.

Instantly I am down on my knees in front of him, my face a foot away from his. I clap my hands together four times, inches from his nose.

"No! No! No! No!" I yell as loudly as I can. Ben's eyes widened, his mouth closed, arrested in mid-scream.

"I know," I say quietly to Ben. "I know. I'm sorry. I'm sorry."

Everyone in the library is looking at us in shock.

Fine. Let the library revoke my privileges. There are other libraries. I have little left to lose except my son, and I will fight for him.

But the terrible power I possessed brought with it a terrible loneliness. I knew that Ben could learn. I was sure he had a shot at recovery. I knew precisely how to teach him. This knowledge separated me from every other human being on the planet, especially from those nearest to Ben. I was dragging him kicking and screaming into the world of normalcy. With one hand tied behind my back.

THE BENJAMIN PROJECT

If no one would help me, I would have to recover Ben myself. I rented a suite in the back wing of Rainbow Apartments, an out-of-the-way, sunny third-floor location where Ben's tantrums would be shielded, I hoped, from the prying eyes of neighbors and Child Protective Services.

Catherine Maurice described the staffing procedure, and it sounded straightforward enough. I was going to need six therapists working in shifts for a total of forty hours a week. Recruit college psychology students. Pay double minimum wage. Train them myself.

I set myself a goal. By noon, I would write six letters to the psychology departments of local universities, asking them to post a help-wanted notice on their bulletin boards.

I wrote out a task list:

1. Look up the universities.
2. Make the mailing list.
3. Address the envelopes.
4. Call the departments.

I froze. This can't possibly work, I thought. The secretary who'd answer the phone would not understand what I was talking about. Your son is what? Autistic? And you want to recover him? Ah-ha-ha-ha-ha-ha-ha. Autistic children don't recover. No, you may not speak to the professor. He is busy. Who is your doctor? You fired your doctor? Are you crazy? This is a university psychology department, not a clinic. You need to call the hospital. We don't see patients here.

She would be right. I was crazy. I dreaded making that first phone call like an execution.

Should I join the Autism Society of America, the hostages, and go listen to the minutes of the last meeting instead of risking this madman's folly? I'd rather be shoveling asphalt than making these calls.

But I picked up the phone, dialed the University of Texas at Arlington, and asked to speak to the chair of the psychology department. What did I have to lose?

Only Ben.

The secretary put me through to Dr. James Kopp.

After three minutes of conversation it was clear that Dr. Kopp was from another planet. Good. Most earthlings hadn't been much help so far. Dr. Kopp had read the Lovaas study. He had even tried to set up a classroom along the lines of the Lovaas experiment but the school district had lost its nerve and pulled the plug.

Would his students be interested in recovering an autistic child?

Yes. Randall Wheeler, Dr. Kopp's top student, was about to graduate and needed a job. He was King of the Rat Lab.

"My parents were weird and I wanted to understand them so I majored in psychology," Randall explained. Patient, deliberate, mature beyond his twenty-two years, he built computers, played the guitar, danced at nightclubs, and trained rats. Whether he was arranging the furniture or drilling Ben, he thought through his next move like a chess player, and he executed the strategy with confidence and grace.

"He's a tyrant," Mom said. "He treats Ben like a machine. The drills! The same words, over and over. Your son is not a laboratory rat!"

I pleaded with her for patience. Mom was paying for the therapy with checks and a legacy from Dad, money that she kept in the fridge, her "cold cash." Seeing is believing, and she could see the results. But she could not be left alone in the apartment with Randall when he was doing language drills with Ben, because she would challenge him with her Freudian analysis. He must have a cold and rejecting father; he must be negating the parental role. Didn't he have any instincts? Why couldn't he give Ben more tender loving care?

Randall explained: "When I am with Ben, I am not a parent, I am a scientist. This is not revenge on my father, this is what I learned in school." Then he would try to show her the data sheets.

"I can't believe you sit there hour after hour and take data on my grandson! What kind of a person are you?"

I didn't care, as long as Randall could potty train Ben. He sat Ben on the toilet and gave him as much juice as he would drink. When Ben peed, Randall rewarded him with an M&M. Then he moved Ben to a chair about a foot away from the toilet and repeated the process. This time, though, when Ben started to pee, Randall picked him up and put him on the toilet seat. Next time, Randall moved the chair two feet away.

The pee training cycle went on all day. I was working in the next room and could hear the toilet flush. Success! I relieved Randall every couple of hours, but Ben got no breaks. By eight o'clock that evening, a dozen six-packs of juice later, Ben was out of the bathroom and into the bedroom, trotting to the toilet as needed.

Randall had accomplished what no one else had been able to do. Though there would be setbacks and we would continue to generalize his training for the next year using overcorrection and positive practice, Ben was essentially potty trained in twelve hours.

&   &   &

I hired six college students to work under Randall as assistant therapists, using discrete trial therapy. Ben made progress, but sometimes the going was rough. Ben resisted.

Ellen, one of Ben's therapists, placed three objects on the table: a book, a shoe, and a sock.

"Ben, look at me," said Ellen. He looked at her. Randall was taking data, writing pluses and zeroes.

"Good looking, Ben." She extended her hand. "Give me book." He pushed a sock toward her. Randall wrote a zero. Ellen put her hand down. Patiently she repeated, "Give me book." She raised her hand expectantly.

The challenge for Ben was discrimination: to learn the difference between words. Learning required effort, work. And he'd been perfecting his work-avoidance strategy for years.

"Give me book," insisted Ellen.

He threw a shoe at her. Randall wrote another zero.

Unruffled, she repeated, "Give me book."

Ben's eyes bulged. He screamed, bit his hand, and threw himself on the floor, kicking, grabbing, and pinching, hitting himself in the face.

Normally I'd have endured the tantrum, waited him out. But that afternoon his performance was convincing. He seemed wracked beyond endurance. Surely he would break a bone or swallow his tongue or his little heart would burst.

I remembered a letter that had to be mailed that very minute and fled the therapy room.

In the car, my illusions crumbled. Ben would never recover. His story would never be told. I should just keep driving, follow the sun. But I had no place to go.

Returning to the therapy room, I wouldn't have been surprised to see ambulance flashers, crime scene tape, Ben—or a therapist—carried out on a stretcher. I was prepared to shut down the program.

But there was no sign of turmoil. In the therapy room, four new objects adorned the table: a bead, a cup, a ball, and a bone.

"Give me cup," said Ellen.

Ben gave her the cup.

"That's ten out of ten," said Randall. He wrote a plus. I looked at the data. Ben was earning top scores.

"What happened?"

"He went on for about twenty minutes," Randall said, "then got up and went to work."

In the spring of 1994, encouraged by the progress Ben was making in his home program, I visited with Sue McBrayer, principal of Walnut Hill Elementary School, to see if Ben's face-to-face sessions could be increased from thirty minutes a day to several hours. I brought with me Lovaas's book, *Teaching Developmentally Disabled Children: The Me Book.* It set off alarms throughout the school district. A week later, on May 16, 1994, I received a letter from Ms. Seevers, Ben's teacher, the one who had introduced me to discrete trial teaching. She explained that aversives, even hand-clapping or a raised voice, which are part of the Lovaas model, are not allowed in the classroom.

"We make an effort to maintain a calm, pleasant, and positive atmosphere in our classroom," she wrote. "We adhere to the model of the TEACCH Program which is used in Total Communication classes throughout the district. We work hard to teach functional communication, appropriate social behaviors, and functional independence skill—all of which are necessary for a child if he is to be integrated into the community." She was referring to the Treatment of Autistic and Communication-handicapped Children program, which competed with Lovaas therapy. I was sure that Ms. Seever's principal had made her write the letter plugging TEACCH, probably dictated it to her.

I called Ms. Seevers at home. "I bought *The Me Book*," I said. "I watched the videos. I taught Ben 'stand up,' 'pat head,' 'touch nose.' I'd like to work with you to recover Ben. I think we can take him all the way through the curriculum."

"Unfortunately," Ms. Seevers said, "I can't work with your son."

"Why?"

"I was fired."

Ms. Seevers explained that the principal had told her that food was not allowed as a reward in the school. Ms. Seevers refused to change the way she taught. It was an impasse.

Had the TEACCH program ever recovered an autistic child?

No. Because autistic children, as nearly everyone believed, do not recover.

As Ben's seventh birthday approached, I felt that we were running out of time. Ben was making good progress at home, but so far we weren't seeing much change in his behavior at school. His gains were confined to the therapy room. We needed to go nuclear.

&ea;   &ea;   &ea;

The challenge in building a nuclear device is the detonator. The fissionable material, uranium, must be instantly compressed to a critical mass, coal into diamond, to trigger the big bang. The solution is to wrap TNT around the uranium. The explosion creates a centripetal force that crushes the uranium core and triggers a nuclear chain reaction. That's what I wanted for Ben—a detonator, a centripetal force that would trigger a recovery.

The detonator, I decided, would be a family intervention: The Benjamin Project. If we could get most of the family focused on Ben for two weeks we could leverage his behavior modification program out of the recovery room and into the real world.

I planned The Benjamin Project to begin in July of 1994. He'd be on the road to recovery by his birthday, when he turned seven.

Dorothy signed on. I sent her a copy of *The Me Book*, and she devoured it. She came down from Iowa to participate in the project, bringing Bay, her big white German shepherd. And Torey, her houseboy.

Mom signed on too and brought her checkbook.

Hannah was out of state for college, going to summer school at Oklahoma State and working at Kinko's. Pete was busy with his job and new family, but offered Dorothy and Torey a place to stay.

The plan hit a snag. Sue was deeply involved in her therapy with Dr. Dunckley, often distracted and self-absorbed, and had little energy or attention available for Ben. She was keeping him part time, though not safely, and was not, as far as I could tell, contributing to his advancement.

"Ben has foreign objects in both ears," I said.

"Why did you tell me?" she replied.

"So we could work together to get them out," I explained.

"Why did you look?" she asked.

Sue had turned away from the pain of Ben's disease, his broken-ness and neediness, which perhaps reminded her of her own. But in my view at the time, she was being a bitch. I told her so, and the altercation turned physical. She refused to talk to me on the phone and she returned my letters unopened: "Return to sender." Her absence was a major blow to the project, but I hoped she would have a change of heart when her mother came to town.

On the eve of the project my doorbell rang. I shoved the vacuum cleaner behind a chair and opened the door. Backlit against the night by the moon and stars was Torey.

"I locked the keys in the car," he said. "Do you have a coat hanger?

Torey and I went dancing at the Village Station, "Boys Town," as he called it. I had a great time.

Next day, Randall and I got down to work. We taught Ben some consonant sounds: *wuh, fuh, puh, muh, tuh, duh.* Put them together and we got *water, food, potty, mama, dada.* He learned to nod yes and no. By the weekend, his attention span had increased and he had become more compliant. Randall's note sums it up: "Ben settled down and initiated work on his own in intervals up to 15 minutes."

The family wasn't much help, though. Each of them brought personal baggage that undermined the project. Dorothy, Mom, and Torey drove endlessly around the cabin of Dallas's founder, where I was supposed to meet them. I was standing behind the Old Red Courthouse. They saw me, but couldn't find a place to park. Mom was in her manic stage. Bay, the white shepherd, was between them, barking. I could hear them yelling at each other.

"Stop!" screamed Mom.

"Shut up, Jeanne," yelled Dorothy.

During the week, Sue confronted her mother for ignoring her father's abuse. Dorothy wanted reconciliation. She met with Sue in therapy, but she cut the session short because, she said, "It's snowing in Iowa," a pathetic excuse to escape. She and Torey planned to drive back to Ames the next day.

I'd had a memorable week, a marker on the journey to recovery, but I didn't get the detonation I was hoping for. Measured against my expectations, the first two weeks of The Benjamin Project fizzled. But it set the stage for later developments. Mom continued to fund therapy and would play an important role in Ben's recovery in years to come.

The last day of their visit, Torey was sitting beside my desk, playing the guitar, while I graphed data on Ben's drills. Torey related well to Ben. He took him on walks around Bachman Lake, introduced him to the neighbors' pets, and showed him how to transplant flowers.

"Why don't you stay and help me raise him?" I asked Torey.

"Because I'd feel all the time the way I feel now," he said. "Torn apart."

That afternoon, Torey and I, just friends, took a goodbye walk around the neighborhood. He was singing and making up lyrics, words like fireflies that blinked off and were lost, blinked on again somewhere else. Baubles.

"My name is Torey," he sang, "and the things I draw come true."

I thought about that song after Torey left, and I wrote him a letter.

"Torey, draw a child who can read, who rides a bicycle, who speaks, who swims," I wrote. "Draw a boy who plays baseball, dials telephone numbers and calls his grandmother; who buttons his shirt, checks out books at the library, writes letters to his Mom and Dad, rows a boat, plays cards and soccer, mows lawns. This is my son to be. Imagine him. Draw him. And then with God's help I will make it happen, one step at a time."

    र   र   र

In the fall of that year, October 11, 1994, I started a new part-time job at the University of Texas in Arlington. I was hired to write a book on the Scenario-based Engineering Process, but in fact I spent most of my time supervising Visual Basic programmers on a Defense Department contract through the university. In my absence from the therapy room, I felt Ben's recovery program needed reinforcements. I applied to the Dallas County Mental Health and Mental Retardation agency for assistance. To qualify, seven-year-old Ben had to be tested. Because we had started his recovery program, I was actually afraid that he might lose his diagnosis and not be eligible for services.

I needn't have worried.

"The client tended to wander around the room aimlessly and periodically grew quite distressed for no apparent reason," wrote the evaluator. "He chewed on the test materials, masturbated on the door and chair, crawled on top of the evaluator as though he were a young infant, burst into sudden bouts of brief screams, and tried to express himself using only primitive verbal grunts and groans."

The report continued relentlessly for ten excruciating pages, but the prognosis section was brief: "The client's difficulties appear to be severe, and it is quite likely that his cognitive capacities, his social inter-actions, his linguistic skills, his ability to use symbolic or imaginative play, will all evidence significant impairment for the life of the child."

I was appalled by this report. But I recognized the behavior as Ben's extreme work-avoidance mode, the pit out of which I was dragging him. Of course Ben was severely impaired, but he was not an idiot. He didn't want to work, and he was conning the evaluator, a con he'd worked with his mother and grandmother for years. In therapy we'd have dealt with it, but the county evaluator was an easy mark. How hopeless Ben appeared to her. How deluded his dad, babbling about recovery.

How many doors have been slammed shut on kids like Ben who have convinced their evaluators that they cannot be recovered?

On the positive side, Ben qualified for services. And if we needed a really low baseline, we had it.

Expect a Miracle

In April of 1995, as Easter approached, I revived my diary. Many of my recollections from this period are based on diary entries.

April 2, 1995. Seven-year-old Ben in tow, I went to a Holy Week healing service with the Reverend Shelley Hamilton, a minister at my church. "Agnes Sanford says, 'Expect a miracle,'" I reminded her. "Where is the miracle?"

"The miracle must happen in you," said Shelley, "and in Ben, and in everyone in your family." She prayed for me, "God, we challenge you. How long will this man have to stand here at this altar in pain?"

With Easter Sunday just days ahead, I struggled with my faith and with my role in Ben's recovery. Mom argued that Ben needed to be placed in an institution. "You've worked with Ben for a year now," Mom said, "poured everything you had to give into him. When others stumbled and fell, you kept going." I agreed with most of her points: that Ben had not recovered; that he needed a consistent environment; that I could not meet all his needs by myself. Sue couldn't do it either.

"I want him to go as far as he can," I said.

"What if he already has?" Mom asked.

"I don't believe it," I said. "I see progress every week."

But she had a point. It was too late to get a full recovery of the kind Catherine Maurice facilitated in her children. Ben evidently belonged among the 52 percent of children in the Lovaas study who improved but did not fully recover. He'd advanced, but I had to agree that he would likely never lose the autistic label, and never be indistinguishable from normal children.

Unless we could ramp his program back up to forty hours per week and keep it there indefinitely. Unless somebody could manage Ben's recovery better than I.

April 3, 1995. About midnight I woke up to Ben's hysterical laughter. He was smearing his feces on the walls, the blankets, his clothes. I gave him a cold shower, got out the bucket and brush, made him clean it up. He wouldn't stop laughing.

I snapped. I slapped him on the back with my open hand. He didn't cry. But he did stop laughing. Frightened and ashamed, I called Dr. Dunckley. "I lost it," I confessed. "I slapped Ben."

"How long have you been working on recovery with him?" Dr. Dunckley asked.

"A year."

"For Ben to revert to a behavior so symptomatic," he said, "would seem to indicate a lack of appreciation for the sacrifices you have made."

Exactly, I thought.

"What's been going on in your life?"

"Grief."

"Your grief indicates there is a loss somewhere," Dr. Dunckley said.

"I'm thinking about going back to work full time," I explained. "But I'm not giving up. I'm planning a full-scale recovery program."

"Who will manage the program?" asked Dr. Dunckley.

I saw in a flash that what I was about to attempt was madness. Catherine Maurice ran a full-scale program. But Maurice had preschool children, a housekeeper, and a husband who supported her both financially and emotionally. I was hoping to achieve the same results, complete recovery, with an older child, as a single parent, no domestic help, no significant financial assets, and a psychotic ex-wife. While I was working full time.

"No one can work full time and run a full-scale recovery program," said Dr. Dunckley.

He was right. Last time I'd ended up kicking holes in the wall.

"You need a vacation, a break," he said. "You need to get something into your life besides Ben."

"That's why I'm going back to work. I'll hire someone to manage the program."

A few days later, Ben and I took a long walk by Bachman Lake. The path was full of children, lovers, families. Ben kept leading me to the lake, and I sat by him and did pat-a-cake and finger plays, thinking about Mom's suggestion, an institution, a "home" for Ben. If a divided house caused the kind of regression I've seen from time to time in Ben—the feces smearing, for example—and if neither Sue nor I could raise him by ourselves, might institutionalization be a better choice?

Logically, yes. He'd done well for a month at Timberlawn.

But the answer wasn't logical. It came welling up from within me like a geyser. I couldn't give Ben away. It felt like betrayal. Ben trusted me to take care of him as I had promised, now and forever.

Shelley says there is no resurrection without a crucifixion. I'd spent years in the tomb. I hoped for a resurrection in Ben's life, and in mine.

April 12, 1995. "I cannot recover Ben," I wrote in my diary. "I cannot run his program and work, and I cannot bear to put him away. Is there no way out of this dilemma?"

That night I dreamed my crew was clearing a path through a jungle. As the leader, I was supposed to guide them through woods, hills, flood, lost towns, and across a lake to an undisclosed location.

I couldn't read the map and couldn't find the path. By contrast, a movie company used a helicopter to cut a swath through the tree branches straight to the destination across the lake and filmed the entire passage with a single tracking shot. All I had to do was get out of the way.

What was this dream telling me? Was I standing in the way of Ben's recovery?

April 14, 1995. On Good Friday, my faith struggle reached a climax, Gabriel on one shoulder, Beelzebub on the other.

GABRIEL. With God as your ally, how can you doubt that you will be successful in recovering Ben?

BEELZEBUB. Because Abba does not cure AIDS sufferers or hurricane victims no matter how hard their parents pray.

GABRIEL. But Abba wills the health and healing of all God's children.

BEELZEBUB. Why then are we not all healed?

Good question, I thought. But suppose we look at it the other way. Not that Abba is my ally, but that I am Abba's ally. In that case my job is not the healing of Ben, but the healing of all creation.

BEELZEBUB. Impossible.

Only from a human perspective.

Before Easter service, Shelley invited us to write on purple strips of cloth what we wanted to get rid of. I wrote, "The belief that Ben's recovery is up to me." As I laid my cloth at the foot of the cross, I prayed, "Abba, take my life, take Ben's life, take his recovery, and make it yours."

I told Mom that I had given Ben's recovery over to God. She assumed I meant I was giving up and was ready to put him in a home. "No," I explained, "I am not giving up. I am letting go."

April 16, 1995. That Easter evening I spent some time working with Ben and enjoyed it. I kept him busy: turn on light, open door, get stool, step up, step down, open, get clothes, put in washing machine, take off lid, pour soap, start machine, say "gum," take off paper, open, throw away, empty dominoes, put away dominoes, put away pennies, on and on, just marching him through the house and having him follow instructions, perform some task at every station. I was surprised and pleased at how cooperative and compliant he was.

"Thank God," I wrote, "that Ben is not dying; that he responds to praise; that he can blow out the candle in 'This Little Light of Mine'; that he does not have an ear infection this month; that he puts on his clothes; that he hasn't had a potty accident for weeks; that he opens the car door, puts in his bag, gets in, and closes the door without having to be instructed on each step; that he stays in his room as a rule after bedtime, even when the door is open; that his eye contact has improved; that he is not in pain; that he enjoys chewing gum."

Thank you, God, who made all things.

In the weeks following Easter 1995, seven-year-old Ben's glow came back. His feelings and thoughts crossed his face like breezes caressing a meadow of flowers, sunlight through drifting clouds. Communication improved. Ben began nodding yes and shaking his head no unprompted in answer to questions. "Ben, do you want cheese?"

Nods yes.

"Ben, are you thirsty? Do you want water?"

Shakes head no.

Later, I gave him a taste of raspberry preserves. "You want more?" I asked. He let the flavor roll around in his mouth.

Penetrating eye contact. A slow, thoughtful nod.

"Now that I can communicate with Ben," I wrote in my diary, "I view him differently and treat him differently. Instead of giving orders I ask questions. This is a watershed development, for Ben and for me."

I wasn't the only one who noticed the change.

"This is weird," said Brett, one of Ben's trainers. He was sitting at a table at Bachman Recreation Center across from Ben.

"I was just talking to him, you know, like I always do," explained Brett. "And I said, 'Ben, you understand me, don't you?' And he, like, looked me right in the eye, and he nodded yes."

"He's been doing that," I observed.

"Then," said Brett, "he smiled and crawled over on me and gave me a big hug."

"Yes, he does that with me too," I said.

"Earlier we were walking," Brett continued, "and I told him to go right. And all by himself he turned to the right."

"Great!"

"Something else is different," Brett continued. "He's smiling a lot. It was actually, like, fun working with him today."

Next day Ben was embracing me, wanting to be lifted and hugged as we walked and cycled along the Bachman trail. Thanks be to God. These are sweet moments and I feel that I cannot savor them enough. I'm still doing discrete trials with him, teaching him, but without the inflexible demands of a few weeks ago. But I work with him respectfully, grateful for the gift of his presence, for the privilege of spending time with him in his short childhood, this uncertain life.

Welcome back, beloved son.

Mom, who had been skeptical of Ben's prospects, came down on the side of the angels. We held hands, and she prayed, "We give thanks for the life of Benjamin Burns, and we know that he is yours. We declare this year a victory."

A victory that would be dwarfed by the struggle ahead.

Progress and Challenges

I'd done my part: set up and run the pilot program, hired six therapists, and facilitated the first difficult year of therapy. I handed the reins of the recovery program to Jon Beckman, a Lovaas-trained consultant. On June 3, 1995, Beckman ran a sixteen-hour workshop for my therapists, then stayed on as project coordinator.

By October 1995, eight-year-old Ben was making stellar scores (80 percent–100 percent) in attention, facial imitation, receptive color, receptive names, building blocks, beads, sorting and picture communication. We planned to follow up with two years of discrete trial therapy, twenty to forty hours per week, then mainstream Ben into the public school system.

At work, I was proud to be associated with a real research university and working on a Defense Department project. The God's Guarantee Committee at our church had been praying that I would be "fully restored" from all my losses. I thought that might be asking a bit too much, but I started saving for a house and I bought medical insurance for Ben and me, thankful for my new position.

Ben's cognitive skills were increasing. I could see him making choices. Which door of the car to get in: front or back? Which side?

He listened, weighed, considered, and decided. "Ben, do you want to go to the children's Christmas service at church?" I asked.

He thought about it for a moment, looked at me, and nodded yes.

I read the Mother Goose book to him. Ben supplied the rhyming word like he did when he was little, before the regression. When I stopped short ("Twinkle, twinkle, little ...") he'd twist his head around like a puppet, look me in the eye, and spit out the missing rhyme word as if he were firing a rifle.

"Stah!"

Janie, one of his therapists, said to me, "He's beginning to talk now. I'm excited. You must be really excited!" I wasn't so much excited as relieved. Ben was becoming more compliant. No more yelling at him or clapping hands in his face in the library or the grocery store.

"Push the cart, Ben." I walked in front of the metal shopping cart, steering it with one hand behind me.

"Good job, Ben. You're a big boy!" He must have felt some sense of control, too. At least he didn't run through the aisles screaming.

As Ben rejoined the human race, so did I. But he continued to challenge me in ways I did not want to be challenged. "He discovers my weaknesses," I wrote in my diary. "He turns my life into boot camp, an obstacle course."

I'd handed the Lovaas program to Beckman, but what about Ben's medical needs? What about leveraging him into the school system? Sue was deeply involved in her recovered memory therapy and wasn't capable of safe and effective parenting. As I saw it, she was essentially babysitting him. The realization sank in: Of all Ben's caregivers, I was the only one who could put the pieces together. "If I don't call The Autism Queen to schedule a re-evaluation," I wrote in my diary, "who will? If I don't demand that the schools provide a free and appropriate education, who will?"

Just getting eight-year-old Ben from place to place is a challenge. We are getting into the car, bound for Bachman Recreation Center and Ben's free swim period. Just enough time to drop him off and get to class. I watch Ben get into the car and pull his clothes bag after him. "Close the door, Ben." *Ca-chunk*. I pull up at Bachman and turn to look in the back seat. No clothes bag, no swimming suit. Maddened, a stuck bull, I spray gravel and careen back to the apartment parking lot. No bag. I lock Ben in the car and dash upstairs. Scuffed as if it had been dragged, his bag is hanging on my apartment door. But I saw Ben put it into the car. No. I saw Ben *start* to put it in the car, and my mind filled in the rest. Why can't I learn to observe, test, check, and not assume anything?

I am too rushed, too stressed.

The problem of time is especially acute in transitions. I prepare to teach my literature class by rereading the assignment and making a list of discussion questions until the very minute that I must leave the house to get to class on time. Then comes the transition. I can change my shirt and pants, comb my hair and pack my books in the fifty-nine seconds it takes me to heat a cup of coffee in the microwave. That very last minute is probably the minute that Ben will go potty in his pants.

My son is making me over. I am impatient; only patience teaches Ben. I value efficiency and speed; Ben requires up to thirty seconds to take off a sock. I value order; Ben destroys his possessions and wrecks his room.

Grandfather Burnsy, the family patriarch, had one memorable piece of advice for me: "To succeed in life, you must make yourself acceptable to other people." But Ben is accepted only by the few people who understand autistic children, and having an autistic son does not elicit understanding in the social and professional circles to which I once aspired.

Other Burns family values were shaped by life before Ben: "Be financially independent." Not likely, unless I inherit wealth. "Don't accept charity." If it weren't for charity, public and private, how would I survive? "Be an achiever. Put your job and career ahead of everything else. Succeed by developing your academic skills; narrow your focus to the written word; seek intellectual challenges." My intellectual challenge today is practical: how to whisk Ben to the toilet before he has an accident, and what clothes to put in the dryer in case he does.

Taking care of my autistic son requires a reversible self, like a reversible coat: turned inside out, Jonathan Edwards, the preacher and dreamer, becomes Benjamin Franklin, the practical man of calendars, shillings, and action. If you'd called me up before Ben and asked me what I was wearing, I'd have to look down at my shirt and pants to tell you. What day is it? A middle-of-the-week day. But when I'm taking care of Ben, I'd better know what day it is. On Wednesdays, he swims at school, so send a towel, swimsuit, and extra underwear, unless the weather is bad. I'd better know where the car is parked unless I want to dash frantically around the Tom Thumb parking lot with a tantrumming kid who needs to use the bathroom. Ben cannot be raised by an absent-minded professor. Taking care of him, recovering him, requires presence of mind and the ability to live fully in the present moment.

Frustrations were building. I was stealing time from my job at UTA to take care of Ben, but there weren't enough hours in the day. One Monday morning I banged the snooze button and slept another hour. Got up just in time, I thought, to get Ben to school and me to work. No more slipping in late.

"Where are the algorithms?" my boss had demanded. The Defense Department was waiting.

"They'll be on your desk 9:00 Monday." *In one hour.*

I dumped Ben's diaper turd in the toilet, showered him, toweled him, chaired him, drenched his red and purple Fruit Loops with milk, and popped a chocolate-coated vitamin B6 into his mouth. He'd been trained to swallow on command. I'd started with a pinch of the horrid yellow goo and worked up to a chocolate-coated pellet, bottle-cap size. Had to be washed down with Kool-Aid, Wacky Wild flavor, squeeze bottle inserted in his puckered lips like an air hose. Where was the Wacky Wild? At the 7-11.

"Swallow!" I bluffed. Ben's cheeks puffed out. Yellow goo trick-led from the corner of his puckered mouth, ran down his chest and dribbled onto his shorts.

Bob Anterhaus, Ben's homeroom teacher, known as Mr. Bob, was not a believer in megavitamins, especially on clothes or carpet. "There!" he'd said on Friday, pointing to a large yellow blot. "And there!" Extending his shoe, he nudged Ben's pillow, a stinky yellow mess that looked like it had been puked out of a garbage disposal.

"Ben needs his B6," I protested.

Mr. Bob was red-faced. "Then he needs to swallow before he comes in here."

By 8:15 that frantic Monday, the Fruit Loops in Ben's bowl were bloating and turning purple. He couldn't eat them with vitamin gunk in his mouth, and he wouldn't spit it out, so we were stuck. I looked at the clock. Time to get him dressed.

Ben's blue shorts were in the clothes hamper, nothing on them but a splash of spaghetti sauce. I scraped it off with my thumbnail and slipped the shorts over his diaper. Yellow goo trickled out of his puckered mouth. If I left now, I could stop at the 7-11 on the way to school, pick up the Wacky Wild, coax the vitamins down Ben, and still get to work on time. I ran down the checklist pinned to his knapsack: towel, swimming suit, underpants, socks, extra shirt, Cheetos, and notebook. I brushed his hair, put on his coat and knapsack. Ready to go.

Oops. Brown paper package on the mantel, a ticking time bomb, waiting for a ride to the post office. Another delay, but I can handle it. I seatbelt Ben, start the car. Gasoline needle brushes the "E." Enough cash in my wallet for Kool-Aid, gas, and lunch? Fourteen dollars, cutting it close. I drive to the 7-11, gas up, and walk down the aisle toward the Kool-Aid.

On days like this there is a tipping point: the morning slides from I-can-handle-this to no-fucking-way. Rain Man's brother, Char-lie, passed this point when he was late to work and Rain Man had to buy his underpants at Kmart. Rain Man wouldn't get on the airplane. Had to watch Judge Wapner. Did not understand that Charlie has obligations, must be at a certain place at a certain time. Isn't the compulsion to be at work on time like the compulsion to buy underpants at Kmart? But other people depend on Charlie, not on Rain Man. I am about to be late for work. The Defense Department is waiting for its algorithms. And I am at the mercy of an autistic child who won't swallow his meds.

My tipping point occurs in the 7-11 when I discover that the Wacky Wild has been replaced by Gatorade. I buy the Gatorade, punch a straw into his mouth, and say "Ben, take a sip." A yellow swirl of gunk descends lazily into the impostor beverage. I seethe at the edge of rage, in need of a good slap. "Idiot," I say to myself. What is Plan B? There is none. But there is a Tom Thumb grocery store a few blocks from Ben's school. Why hadn't I thought of that sooner?

I check my watch, step on the gas. Ben's class is having breakfast now, and I'm driving forty miles per hour though a school zone. Fine. If I'm arrested I'll just make the cop shoot me. Pulling into the Tom Thumb parking lot, I consider leaving Ben in the car while I run in for the Kool-Aid. Bad idea. If I get stuck in a checkout lane, Ben could jump out of the car and run into the traffic. I'll have to take him with me.

I get out of the car, walk around to Ben's side, and open his door. That's his cue to unbuckle his seatbelt and get out. He does nothing. "Unbuckle," I say. He does nothing. We have rehearsed this behavior dozens of times, but never with B6 in his mouth. "Ben, get out," I scream. He does nothing.

What now? I am past the tipping point, unglued, Evel Knievel missing the leap. I could call my boss and tell him I'm not coming in. But if I can't work, I think illogically, what's the good of having a job? I might as well quit. But if I quit, who will pay for Ben's medical insurance? Since I'd gone to work for the university, Ben's health care was on my ticket. The rage comes again, and this time I give into it. I smash the Gatorade bottle onto the asphalt and grab Ben's arm, yelling "Get out of the fucking car, goddamn it!" The worst thing I could do. Knowing this makes me even angrier.

Ben looks at me with frightened, questioning eyes, his mouth puckered, holding in the dissolved B6. All he has to do is swallow it. I am down on my knees in front of him. "Just swallow it, baby. Please."

He does nothing.

I throw him over my shoulder and dump him into a squeaky shopping cart. The automatic door is maddeningly slow. I pound my way through the gap and careen around the store, cart shrieking like a rusty gate. A clerk looks up at me from her perch at the cash window. "Can I help you?"

No, I am beyond help. I plunge toward a knot of customers in the aisle, Dallas Cowboy quarterback Troy Aikman breaking the defensive line. My cart bumps a stack of liquid detergent. Soap bottles scatter like billiard balls. I reach the Kool-Aid section, grab a pack of Wacky Wild, and head for the check out stand. First good break of the day: the line is short. I rip out a Wacky Wild bottle, twist the top off, slip it into Ben's mouth, squeeze. He swallows beautifully, just as he has been trained to do. *Thank you, Abba.*

Driving to Ben's school, I spy the brown paper package waiting to be mailed. I roll up the windows and scream in pain and rage. Better than running down a pedestrian. Or plowing into a whole gaggle of them, I think gleefully, watching them scatter like soap bottles.

Rain Man, at the end of the movie, went back to the institution. Much as his brother Charlie loved him, wanted to keep him, Rain Man didn't belong in the outside world. He had no concept of work, of being late, of a larger, interrelated world with parts that must somehow mesh. Neither did Ben. "Either I must recover my son," I wrote, "dedicate my life to his care, or give him up." Reading these histrionics ten years later, I think: Why didn't I just get up earlier?

        &   **&**   **&**

Back in my graduate student days, when I was learning to fly, I piloted my first cross-country flight in turbulent air, battered like a racquetball between cutthroat players. My little Cessna 150 shot up 200 feet. Wind shear pounded me down to the bottom of the air pocket. I blasted up, crashed back. Each shot left the plane in a frightening orientation: horizon twisted sideways like a broken leg. The map tumbled from my lap and I groped for it, afraid to glance down. I gripped the yoke like a jackhammer.

I should have known, logically, that I was in no real danger. The airplane was built to withstand these forces and once out of the turbulence would return automatically to straight and level flight. But I was out of control, disoriented, head beaten against the ceiling, plunging over the falls. This wasn't the time for logic; this was the time for stark raving fear.

Raising Ben is like that. I remove a pencil eraser from Ben's nose. He stuffs a Snoopy Band-Aid into his sinus cavity. Estimated cost of surgical removal: $2,000, which I don't have. The school calls. Ben has another ear infection, the sixth in eight months. I've had it. I was not brought up to raise an autistic child. But who else will do it?

In late October of 1995, writing to my autism e-mail list, I scribbled myself into a frenzy.

"I'm going to have to pull the plug on Ben," I rant. "I can no longer stand these regressions, these bus plunges. He is recovering from his ear infection. But he will get another one, and I am powerless to prevent it."

I take a deep breath, which I'm going to need. "Four or five sets of ear tubes, a world-famous eye, ear, nose, throat doctor, endless antibiotics, Nystatin therapy, three allergists, allergy shots, hypoallergenic diet, auditory training, consultation with four prayer sessions by a New Age M.D," I continue, piling it on. "Then, WHAM! Ben forgot his colors, numbers, letters, objects. His sleep is chaotic, his language disintegrated, his compliance non-existent. A year's work, wiped out."

"I am bailing out, Ben," I rave on. "I cannot help you. God forgive me my blindness and ignorance, for I know I can never forgive myself. If I could trade places with you, I would!"

Feeling better, I title this e-mail "I Quit" and send it off to my autism e-mail list and Ben's doctor. *The ball is in your court, Abba.*

The next morning at Sunday service, the sermon hit me between the eyes: "Don't Quit." I took notes. The preacher made three points:

1. *People tend to quit just before victory.* Yep. Sue and I did that the first time Ben cratered.

2. *Let go of old baggage.* Someone with a batting average of 400 is a highly sought after hitter, yet he strikes out six times out of ten. If we are to succeed, we must forget the strikeouts and come to the plate fresh.

3. *When you need a friend, call on Jesus.* The third point was a problem for me: I had never been much for calling on Jesus, preferring to bypass the second-in-command and go straight to the top. But in desperate times, I'd had the experience of turning my life and will over to God, of allowing myself to be guided minute by minute until the situation improved. When I left myself open for surprises, I found myself doing surprising things.

I checked my e-mail. I had six responses from my autism e-mail list, all of them with comforting words and practical advice. Reading those parents' posts thirteen years later, I am impressed by their wisdom and foresight. "What helped Alex was putting him on a strict gluten-free and reduced-casein diet," wrote one mother. She also suggested taking Ben off antibiotics. "Aggressive, irritable, goofy, spacey, no learning," she wrote. "That pretty much is what Alex has been like since Amoxil."

Today, I see that the cause of Ben's regressions was not the ear infections, but the antibiotics and the candida overgrowth they triggered, plus Ben's undisciplined diet. How I resisted that insight. But I took comfort from the understanding words of another parent:

"You are not pulling the plug. You are looking ahead, looking for some clear avenue on a very treacherous road."

So much of that road remained to be traveled. But I had volunteered for this, and I wasn't through yet. There were more twists around the bend.

SUE, ME, AND BEN

I visited Tyler State Park to hike in the Piney Woods with Ben and Sue. Though we were divorced, Sue and I still enjoyed occasional family outings together. Sue brought camping gear, a tent, a backseat full of sleeping bags, pillows, blankets, black trash bags erupting with Tupperware, tin foil, and bean cans. That evening, seated beside the campfire, I played the guitar while Ben foraged for food and drank my Coke. Sue read him some stories, played telephone with him. She was relating to him well, becoming more behavioral in her approach. We had a lovely time.

"Would you like to stay the night?" Sue asked.

No thanks. I had plans.

Driving back to Dallas, I couldn't shake the image of holding Ben's hand while we walked down the park road, his head bent back to see the tops of the towering pines, face awestruck. I should have stayed. What plans, what task could be more important than healing my poor, broken little family?

I decided to spend more time with Sue.

The Christmas holiday of 1995, Sue, Ben, and I went to visit Sue's family, in New Orleans, where Sue's mother, Dorothy, and her domestic partner, Mary, had retired. Eight-year-old Ben, our first evening there, was on his best behavior. He sat attentively and took instruction well, I thought. Except he refused to flush the toilet.

"Flush the pot, Ben," I commanded. He ran out of the bathroom squealing. The sound of a flushing toilet triggered his hyperacute hearing and frightened him.

"He had this wry look on his face," said Mary. "He was not going to flush that pot."

Mary, or Dr. Mary Rohrberger, who had been my Ph.D. advisor, had long taken a dim view of Ben. Years before, during Sunday dinner at Dorothy and Mary's rural Oklahoma estate, their homestead on Lost Creek Bluff, two-year-old Ben had made a huge mess, eating tomatoes out of the salad bowl with his fingers, grabbing dessert off Hannah's plate, and setting his drink down half off the table, where it was sure to tumble. And it did. The ill-mannered little miscreant was table-banished; Sue and I, delinquent parents, were disgraced. Sue took Ben to the front lawn, sat him naked in a high chair, garden hose handy for the cleanup, and fed him slices of watermelon until he was covered with seeds and pink juice dripped from his elbows. Mary stalked out of the house to toss leftover salad to the birds. She spied Ben, watermelon slice crowning his head, and stared in horror the way onlookers gawk at a gruesome automobile accident, mesmerized by the junk-strewn impact crater. What could possibly be more appalling? A little arc of pee spurted from Ben's naked lap. Mary shook her head. I knew what she must be thinking: What in the name of God have we wrought.

Mary expected me to achieve a tenured professorship, like hers, or failing that, to make my fortune in business. But Ben had changed me. My ambitions had shrunk. My goal that Christmas was to teach Ben to balance a wooden block on its end and to put the final "t" on "I want that." Mary was not in tune with the new agenda and had little patience with me, Sue, or Ben. She believed that he was autistic because he was angry, and that we need to stop coddling him and "break through the anger."

Early during our Christmas visit, Ben had thrown a tantrum. "Have you considered institutionalizing him before he gets much bigger?" said Mary. "I'm not used to being around a child who is undisciplined." That hurt, because there was some truth in it. Ben was undisciplined because he was living in two households, and the rules were different in each. We needed a more consistent approach, a single set of rules consistently enforced, as they had been at Timberlawn. If I could just get the family back together under a single roof, I thought, Sue and I could recover Ben.

The obstacles to reconciliation were formidable. I was gay and Sue was suffering from a psychological disorder, post-traumatic stress syndrome. In recovered memory therapy, she had recalled that she had been abused as a child. Over time, she had pieced together a narrative in which Dorothy had taken Mary into her bedroom and had moved Susan's dad, Boyd, in with five-year-old Susan. Susan was subject to sexual assaults by her father from age five to fifteen, when Dorothy and Mary moved to Stillwater so Mary could take the job at OSU. Sue had no coherent memory of these assaults because the memories were held by personality fragments—"multiple personalities"—that didn't communicate with each other. In psychological terms, Sue dissociated. She was shattered, broken into tiny pieces. It was her way of handling the pain.

Having known and loved Dorothy, and respecting Mary, I was slow to accept this narrative as essentially true. But evidence of Sue's dissociative disorder was more and more difficult to ignore. Preparing for Ben's allergy test, Sue told me that she had discarded her overstuffed furniture and sprayed her carpet with an anti-allergen pet spray from Eckerd Drugs. When Ben's test came back positive for dust mites, she asked me, "What can you do about it?"

"Spray."

"Spray what?"

"The anti-allergy stuff you got at Eckerd. To neutralize the dust mites."

"I didn't tell you about that," she said. "What is it?"

"You told me you sprayed your carpet."

"No I didn't." She was adamant. "That wasn't me. I never said that."

A miscommunication? In the past, I would have thought so. Sue was so resolute, so certain. I would have questioned my own memory, even my own sanity. But incidents like this one occurred often enough that I began to accept that her diagnosis, Dissociative Identity Disorder, later reclassified as Post-Traumatic Stress Disorder. Evidently, she really was a multiple personality. She had a name for one of her alter egos: The White Bitch. The Rottweiler.

In the film *Unstrung Heroes*, the loving mother, played by Andie MacDowell, is stricken with ovarian cancer. Her little son asks, "Are you dying."

"Yes," she answers. "I'm so sorry." It moved me deeply.

Like the MacDowell character, Sue wanted to be a good mother. But she was in the throes of her illness, and she could not function as she had before. Dr. Dunckley, her psychotherapist, had advised me that, if she undertook recovered memory therapy, she would get worse before she got better. How much worse he didn't say. Once the memories surfaced, she became someone I didn't recognize: Mrs. Hyde. She could not do the things one might expect a mother to do, such as keeping her apartment clean. At the bottom of her descent into psychosis, when she was hospitalized, there was jelly and mustard smeared on the cabinets, rat poison poured like salt into the corners, rice and peas strewn across the living room rug, roaches crawling the walls. There was no hot water. The dishwasher was broken. So was the upstairs window, where Ben crawled out onto the roof. The apartment smelled like a garbage dump except when it filled up with gas from the unlit pilot light. She lost Ben in the Salvation Army store; the police found him blocks away and called me. When I phoned her, she didn't know he was missing.

Shouldn't I be doing for Sue what she cannot do for herself, keep her living quarters clean, safe, and decent? I visited her once a week, took the knobs off the stove so she wouldn't blow herself up, took out the trash and tried to clean up a little. Wouldn't I change her bedpans if she were physically ill?

After Sue's memories of sexual abuse started surfacing in 1991, her fear of her father, who had been dead since the mid-1970s, haunted our relationship. Years later I saw firsthand the fear these rape memories wreaked upon her. Three o'clock in the morning, Sue was downstairs. I heard her crying and went down to comfort her. She was flat on her back in a trancelike state. She was using the muscle massager, a therapeutic device, to trigger body memories so she could bring them to the surface and move them out. I sat down on the floor beside her as she wept. I put my hand on her shoulder. She turned her head, looked at me, and screamed. I thought that the scream was a startle response, that she would recognize me and stop screaming. But she didn't stop. She locked eyes on me and kept screaming, terror on her face. I dropped my eyes and spoke to her gently: "It's OK, it's OK."

At last the trance was broken. "I thought you were my father," she explained. "He threatened to kill me."

If I'd had any doubt about the reality of her flashbacks or the depth of her terror, this experience settled it. Sue was in the grip of fear—haunted, hunted, tormented, hallucinatory, possessed. She was a prisoner of her past, the Auschwitz of her childhood. Yet I could not recover Ben without her.

If Ben were to recover, I was convinced that Sue must recover. While we were married, she was relatively stable. If she spent more time with me, I thought, perhaps even lived with me, she would stabilize again.

I concocted a strategy to win her back. I started cooking good, hearty dinners: homemade chili or roast beef with stewed vegetables. She'd stay for dinner, then she began to do some laundry at my apartment, leaving her clothes around, hanging her bleach-stained red dress on the living room wall, marking her territory. At first the bras and pantyhose were alien, intrusive, like rattlesnake skins. Then I got used to them. Then I got to where I liked having them around.

Sue spent Wednesday and Friday nights at my apartment. I told her little about my life—only what she needed to know—and asked little about hers. Sitting in the old brown grandfather chair, she read a story to Ben. Seeing her close up under the warm incandescent light, hearing again her joking voice, I felt a great tenderness toward her, and a great sadness. I still loved her. But love wasn't enough to tame the anger I felt when Sue behaved irrationally in ways that I felt eroded Ben's progress.

One evening Sue came to my apartment to drop off eight-year-old Ben but wouldn't stay, even for a minute, to discuss some needed changes in his schedule. "Sue, please!" I'd called after her as hurried down the stairs.

"I'm late," she yelled back. "I've got to go. "

"When are we going to talk?"

"I don't know. I'm late."

We'd agreed that Ben should stay here with me during potty training in order to maintain consistency in his environment, but she'd reversed the decision. The next evening, she announced she was taking Ben home with her.

"Tonight is my night, " said Sue.

"He's in potty training," I argued. "We talked about this."

She called the police. "Tonight is my night to take my son," she told them, "and my ex-husband won't let me have him."

"At least wait until I've given him his medication," I said.

"I'll wait outside." She walked away.

I took my time giving Ben his meds. I thought she'd left. Then I heard her say, "I'm leaving now." She had been hanging around the door just out of sight like a child who has threatened to run away but is waiting to be confronted. Hours later the police came. Sue hadn't given them my address. They'd traced the call.

Week after week, pointless arguments continued. "Why didn't you buy him a table that the trainers could sit at?" said Sue, pointing to Ben's expensive new desk-and-chair set. I should have been expecting an attack like this. It was Thursday evening, Sue's therapy day. She was generally on the attack after therapy.

"Why didn't *you*?" I countered.

"I did," she said.

"Good."

"But it's at my house," she continued.

"OK," I acknowledged. I didn't like the tone of this conversation.

"So why didn't you buy him one that the trainers could sit at?" she continued relentlessly. The question struck me as useless, hostile, antagonistic. In a more relaxed mood I might have tried to answer it, but tension had been building all week. It seemed to me that Sue didn't want an answer; she wanted a fight. I gave her the finger.

"Bastard."

"Bitch."

She held up a green pistol grip with a key ring attached to it and pointed it at me. Mace.

"Great idea, Sue. I'd love to have a reason to file assault charges."

She sprayed me in the face. It hit me on the cheek and lips, burned like hot pepper. Good thing I had my glasses on.

Altercations like these came out of nowhere, set back my plans for a domestic relationship. Why did the table have to be an issue? Why couldn't Sue and I just get along?

And what effect were our constant arguments having on Ben?

&a. &a. &a.

I planned to ramp up the training schedule again, go full scale. The previous year I'd aimed for forty hours a week, but with the students' ever-changing schedules and summer vacation, that had slipped from thirty to twenty to ten.

I hoped to bring Sue into the project. When she was at her most sensible and we were focused on the same goals, we accomplished most of them. But her chronic physical frailties and her mental anguish, her PTSD, had made her an unreliable project partner. Could that change?

I went to a meeting of FEAT, Families for Effective Autism Treatment. Sue canceled at the last minute. Linda Mayhew, the founder, had some eye-opening advice. "Many families in our group are going through separation or divorce," she said. "My husband refused to be involved in the autism therapy or in my work with FEAT. At first I was angry. Then I learned that each spouse chooses his or her role. Don't judge. Respect each other for the roles you choose, and be thankful."

What was Sue's role? She provided respite for me. She made home-cooked meals for Ben. When he was an infant, she gave him her undivided love, and even in the midst of her turmoil, she never stopped loving him. Autistic children often don't display affection, but Ben is an exception. Sue lit the lamp of love in him. What greater gift could she have given? That night I wrote, "I am thankful for Sue's love of Ben. I understand that recovery depends not on me, not on Sue, but on the One who makes a way when there is no way, the One who is making all things new."

Later that week Sue and I met at the hospital. Ben was scheduled for surgery to remove a bobby pin from his nasal cavity. Earlier extractions included paper wads, beads, and a Band-Aid. Ben would try to remove objects he'd stuffed in his nose, but his attempts jammed them further in.

"Do you think we'll ever recover? You, Ben, me?" I asked Sue.

"Yes," she said. She was thoughtful for a while. "What do you have to recover from?"

"Total collapse," I answered. "My family, my business, my career. Everything I worked for." For the first time in years she put her hand on mine.

That evening, Sue was sick with the flu and thought she was dying. She asked me to spend the night with her.

"I'm sorry for all the bad things that happened," she said.

"What things?"

"Too many to list," she said.

She asked me what I thought she had accomplished with her life. I thought of the poetry readings she was giving in the Arts District. "You are developing talents and skills you didn't know you had, " I answered.

"So what?" she asked. Then she added, "But we did raise two fine children."

I would have said three.

That night, Sue agreed to share an apartment with me as part of Ben's recovery program.

DOCTORS TO THE RESCUE

"I practice three kinds of medicine," said Dr. Constantine Kotsanis, gesturing, "right, left, and center. On the right, drugs and surgery. On the left, energy fields, prayer, and spiritual healing. The center is nutrition, tests, amino acids, pharmaceuticals when you need them. What kind of treatment do you want for Ben?"

Dr. Kotsanis was an integrative physician and a founding member of Defeat Autism Now!, a society of doctors who pioneered the biomedical approach to treating autism. We had come to enroll Ben in a study that later would become part of the Defeat Autism Now! biomedical protocols, designed to help recover autistic kids.

"We live in a marvelous age," said Dr. Kotsanis. "Libraries at our fingertips. Cell phones in our pockets. Airplanes to France, Athens, Madrid. Call anybody, go anywhere." He looked at me. "So who pays"? He turned around and pointed to Ben. "*He* pays."

Dr. Kotsanis's argument was that toxic waste in our air, food, and water had reached a critical threshold. Autistic kids were canaries in a coal mine. The difference between organized crime and organized medicine was one of degree. HMOs were driven by greed, doctors in the pocket of the drug companies. But no one was blameless.

"Take a gang killing," said Dr. Kotsanis, who hailed from the North Side of Chicago, Al Capone's back yard. "Who is responsible?

The hit man pulls the trigger. But what about the chauffeur? The bag-man? The boss?" Just so, he concluded, we are all responsible for the damage our toxic environment had done to Ben and countless others. Autism, ADD, ADHD were manifestations of an underlying disease. One child in one hundred and fifty, by the government's count, was on the autistic spectrum. One in fifty by Dr. Kotsanis's estimation.

"What about Ben's ear infections?" I asked. We were here for a cure, not a lecture. "The antibiotics aren't helping."

"Of course not," Dr. Kotsanis said. "Antibiotics kill the normal gut flora. Yeast overgrows the gut like weeds and creates neurotox-ins that poison his brain. When you give antibiotics, you should control the yeast with an antifungal, such as Nystatin, and not just locally but systemically. Then you should give probiotics to replace the beneficial flora you killed."

"But what about Ben's ear infections?" I asked.

"His problem is milk."

This doctor is crazy, thought I. Ear infections are caused by germs, which need to be killed. "That's what you've been trying to do for the last ten years," observed Dr. Kotsanis. "Has it worked?

"My grandfather owned a creamery," I countered illogically.

"So did mine," trumped Dr. Kotsanis.

"Then you should know that milk is good for babies," I argued, "good for everybody. Nature's most nearly perfect food."

"That's what the dairy industry wants you to think. They paid for you to think that."

Dr. Kotsanis turned us over to his nutritionist, Jana, who ex-plained that gluten, a component of wheat, was harmful to many autistic children. So was casein, the protein in milk. Jana ran on about enzymes, amino acids, and methylation cycles until my eyes glazed over. She recommended putting Ben on a gluten-free, casein-free (GF/CF) diet. I'd heard that advice before, but I'd resisted. Wheat and milk are key to every meal. Live without bread and cheese? You might as well try to drive without gasoline. But Sue put Ben on a gluten-free diet, and we agreed to eliminate, or at least reduce, his milk and cheese.

⅛   ⅛   ⅛

More help was coming on the medical side. Bill McKnight, a physician assistant, became my counselor and friend. He had an academic's respect for knowledge, research, and problem solving. I made copies of research articles for him. He read them, discussed them with me, did his homework, and tried new therapies on Ben. I'd sent Bill a copy of my "I Quit" letter. He saw it for what it was: a cry for help.

"We need to take another look at Ben," said Bill. "We need to look at all the systems, the whole kid." I agreed. I had confidence that Bill and I could put our heads together and come up with solutions.

Autism had long been considered a psychological disorder, then an untreatable neurological one. But Bill and I were beginning to understand that autism is a treatable, multi-organ disease that involves the gut and the immune system as well as the brain. One of the articles I shared was by Dr. Sudhir Gupta: "Dysregulated Immune System in Children with Autism: Beneficial Effects of Intravenous Immune Globulin on Autistic Characteristics." Gupta had demonstrated that IVIG treatment resulted in improved eye contact, speech, and behavior.

I had not truly grasped that Ben's ear infections could be a *cause* of Ben's autistic behaviors, not just a co-symptom. Like many other parents and all but a few doctors, I never made the link. But Bill suggested that the ear infections might be part of the underlying disorder. Maybe, Bill reasoned, IVIG would reduce Ben's ear infections, and autism would loosen its grip.

Bill went into action. He wrote to Ben's insurance company, documented his medical history. United Health Care would not pay for autism, but they did agree to partially fund the off-label therapy for Ben's ear infections: twelve immunoglobulin infusions, one per month for a year.

When Sue, Ben, and I were waiting at the hospital for the first infusion, I taught Ben how to use the electric up-and-down switch on the examining chair. For the first time Sue witnessed a teaching demonstration, Lovaas therapy at work "Oh, you really taught him something," she said. Years, earlier, she'd closed her door on the therapy because she thought it was abusive. But that day in the hospital, she wasn't being sarcastic. She was coming around.

The IVIG treatment required that Ben be connected to an infusion set for about two hours. He wouldn't hold still. It took five adults to subdue him and strap him to a papoose board. Sue couldn't abide it. She left. By the third infusion, Ben had learned to tolerate the procedure, cooperate, and hold still without being strapped to a papoose board.

The nurse seemed to think that what we were doing for Ben was a misuse of resources. Human immunoglobulin was precious. Like spare body parts, IVIG was scarce and rationed. The waiting list included military hospitals. Its use in treating autism had not been approved, and the risks were significant. Some months, infusions had to be delayed until a supply could be found. The good news: combined with his reduced casein and gluten-free diet, IVIG therapy worked for Ben. For the first year following the infusions, his ear infections were reduced from about one per month to zero.

Ben At School

On the home front, Ben was making good progress in his discrete trial program. He'd mastered catch and throw ball, flush toilet, hang up coat, stack dominoes, chain paper clips, blow up balloon, fold wash cloth, pour water, nod yes and no, spin quarter, empty trash, hang up picture, kick ball, and zip pants.

He'd also learned to imitate the vowel sounds in *saw, see,* and *up,* and the consonant sounds *M, S, F, Wh, B,* and *P.* My student therapists were rehabilitating him like a polio victim, restoring his atrophied neurological system.

Best of all, he had learned to imitate. I could show Ben what I wanted him to do—make a fist, stick out his tongue, cover his head with a blanket—and he would do it. He no longer needed food as a reward: "Good job, Ben!" was reinforcement enough for him. I was confident that he could learn anything we had the patience to teach him. At age eight, he was ready, I thought, for school.

But I was apprehensive about the Dallas Independent School District. They'd fired the only teacher who'd made a breakthrough with Ben. When I picked him up or dropped him off, I often stayed for a few minutes to observe and to chat with the pupils. Jason, a bright, attractive boy, about a year older than Ben, was bouncing on a foot trampoline.

"Jason, sit still," the teacher said.

"No no no no no!" he replied, wiggling away. Wow, the kid could talk.

"Jason, say 'Cookie,'" I prompted.

"Cookie!"

"Good talking, Jason," I said, reinforcing.

"Oh, don't tell him that," the teacher snapped. "He doesn't know what he's saying. He's echolalic." She pronounced the technical term as if explaining nuclear fission to a layperson. In her mind, "echolalic"—meaning he echoed words without understanding them—was a verdict that sealed Jason's fate. She was proud of her master's degree in special education.

I thought Jason's echolalia was a gift. It provided a huge repertoire of sounds that could be shaped into meaningful speech. Jason looked at me with eager eyes. "Save me," his eyes seemed to beg. "Teach me." I taught him to raise arms and clap hands. Ben had needed several lessons to learn those behaviors; Jason learned instantly. His teacher was alarmed. "Extended School Year is for maintenance only," she said. "We're not supposed to teach anything new."

The speech therapist trundled in, late, hauling a heavy institutional tape player that looked like it had been trolled from the back of a storage shed. She arranged five children in a semicircle, fumbled with the tape player, found the right button. *If you're happy and you know it, pat your knees,* instructed the lyrics. Nobody was patting knees. She turned up the volume. Alex hit himself in the face. Jason spun a truck wheel. Ben put his fingers in his ears. Kendall tried to escape. The therapist ignored the kids, chatting with Ben's homeroom teacher.

"Pat your knee, Ben," I said. I mimed a knee pat for him, and he followed the example. "Great!" This was a triple play for Ben: imitation, following instructions, participation. He looked pleased with himself. I expected the therapist to say, "Good patting knee," but she ignored him.

Kendall scooted to the tape recorder and pushed a button. "No, leave it alone," the therapist commanded. "No no no no," said Jason. Kendall pushed another button. The therapist gave up, let him have his way with it. "Don't break it," she ordered. Jason decided to push buttons, too.

Here was an opportunity, I thought, to teach the kids "push button." But the therapist was explaining to the homeroom teacher how long ago she had requisitioned the tape player, how surprised she was when she actually got it, and how sternly she had been instructed to return the ancient, dusty contraption in the same condition that it had been received. So passed the weekly fifteen-minute speech therapy session. It must have been agony for the hapless therapist. It was for me.

Next day I saw Jason's mother at Bachman Recreation Center, where she had come to pick him up. I was excited about the imitation set I'd taught him, keen to show off his learning.

"Jason, look at me," I said. He looked. "Raise arms," I said.

"Jason can't do that," declared his mother.

"Yes he can," I countered. I raised my arms, and Jason raised his. "Do this," I said. I clapped. Jason clapped. But his mother took it badly.

Jason was wiggling out of the seat, trying to run away. "Jason, sit still!" I said. He sat still. His mother hunched over him protectively.

"Jason can't sit still," she said. Jason started wiggling again. She gave him a cookie, rewarding him for proving her right.

That night I received a phone call from Jason's father. He and his wife, he told me, had suffered many terrible disappointments. They'd tried home schooling, but it hadn't worked. They'd moved from Atlanta to Dallas to participate in the school district's TEACCH program. His wife would prefer that I not try to teach Jason anything. She did not want him disturbed.

Perhaps Jason's mother was a model of the people for whom the school system "worked." Nothing could be done, so nothing would be done. Hope was too painful for this suffering mom, and too late for poor, eager Jason.

❧   ❧   ❧

On January 9, 1996, it was time for Ben's regular three-year as-sessment, held at E. D. Walker, a large, two-level decommissioned elementary school in a depopulating area of Dallas. Downstairs: fluorescent lights, photocopiers, cubicles, telephones, and a few computers. I was outside the front door, early, doing body-part drills with Ben, warming him up for the test.

"Touch eyes, Ben." He touched his eyes. "Good. Touch nose."

"May I help you?" said a voice, interrupting. It was one of Ben's teaching assistants. Her tone was anything but helpful.

"Yes, you can help me teach Ben his body parts."

"I don't see a little boy who needs to learn his body parts," she said. "I see a little boy who needs a hug." To me her comment rep-resented the problem with special education in Dallas: low expec-tations. Ben could learn, but he needed rigorous instruction and practice, not coddling.

Upstairs, the carpets were new, walls freshly painted. Balancing a Styrofoam coffee cup that seemed oddly out of place, I walked down the hall to the antechamber of the Autism Queen. There was a play rug on the floor, train tracks, highways, bridges, cars. I set Ben down on the rug, spilling a little coffee. "Vroom, vroom, Ben. Big truck. See? Your turn." He ignored the truck, climbed up one of the chairs and began masturbating. *Not a good start.*

The Autism Queen opened the door to her office. "We'll be ready for Ben in a moment, Mr. Burns." I was trying to keep Ben calm and focused. Jill Varley, the Autism Queen's assistant, perfectly coiffured, swept into the antechamber.

"Hi, Ben. Would you like to play a game?" Ben raised his hand and wrapped it around Ms. Varley's finger. "Wait here, Mr. Burns."

"OK," I said. Ben walked trustingly into the testing room. I bowed my head and made the sign of the cross. Though I wasn't Catholic, I'd picked up the habit from my Catholic friends. But I couldn't remember whether to go right to left or left to right.

Ten minutes later the door opened and Ms. Varley stuck her head out, brushing her hair from her face. "Mr. Burns, will you come in here, please." The testing room felt ten degrees hotter than the waiting room. Ben was sitting at a table facing a large bureau mirror, emotionally zoned out and hitting himself on the chin.

"Ben, look at me," I said. But he wouldn't take his eyes off the mirror.

"Let's turn him around," I said. We moved the table out from the mirror and set Ben with his back to it. "Quiet hands, Ben," I said. Ben put his hands in his lap. Ms. Varley had some wooden blocks in front of her, different shapes, sizes, and colors. She was giving Ben the Brigance Inventory of Basic Skills, the test that he had done so miserably on three years earlier.

"Ben, I'm going to put the blue block over here," she said, "and I want you to match the color." Ben picked up the blue block and put it in his mouth. She looked at me for help.

"Ben, put with same," I said, using a key phrase. He put the blue block on the blue square as he had been trained. He just hadn't understood her instructions. "Put the blue block with the other blue blocks" meant nothing to him; he could only respond to key phrases. But I couldn't be at Ben's side to translate for him every day.

I received the written evaluation a few days later. Ben's performance was awful. He chewed on the test materials, threw them on the floor, slapped the table, shook his hands, tensed his body, hyperventilated, and tried to pull Ms. Varley's hair. On adaptive skills he scored one year, four months. On imitation, perception, and fine motor skills, he did no better than a two-year-old, same as on the previous test, three years earlier.

"How did it go?" Sue asked.

"His IQ tested 28," I replied.

That was in the very severe range of mental retardation, idiot territory. But I knew that Ben was no idiot. We'd worked on his Brigance skills in therapy, and he could perform most of the intermediate tasks in the 80–90 percent range. In the therapy room. With his therapists. But his new skills needed to be generalized to the classroom, then to the real world.

We had our work cut out for us.

🐌   🐌   🐌

Exercising my right as a parent, I called a meeting of Ben's Admission, Review, and Dismissal committee. In an ARD, as the meetings are called, administrators, teachers, and parents develop an Individual Education Plan (IEP), including goals, for each child. By default, the teacher makes recommendations and the parents approve, but there are thirty to fifty pages of paperwork that must be filled out. It's a little like a court procedure. Administrators attend the meeting to make sure all the system rules, numerous and arcane, known only to ARD committee experts, are not violated. Anyone in the ARD can call out, "You didn't say 'may I,'" and everybody has to take three steps back. ARDs can be disorienting and disheartening to parents, who may feel powerless. Jargon, acronyms, and innumerable rules conceal the school's helplessness. By accident, I learned that parents *do* have power.

In March of 1996 the ARD committee, responding to my request, met to discuss Ben's three-year evaluation and to adjust his IEP. Ben's ARD goals were to increase vocalizations, attention span, and cooperation.

Same as at the last ARD, and the one before that, but there was no quantification, no specificity, no accountability, no teaching plan. No one in the system, I thought, understood how to teach these kids. How was Ben's progress going to be measured, and how would we know when his goals were achieved?

I'd written a letter to Ben outlining my expectations of him. I'd asked that these instructional objectives be incorporated in Ben's February 7, 1995, IEP. The committee had agreed. Some items from that list, which went on for several pages:

Don't tear up your books.
If you drop something, pick it up.
If you spill something, clean it up.
If you open something, close it.
If you turn something on, turn it off.
When you finish playing with a toy, put it away.
Learn fingers: pointer, tallman, ringman, pinkie.
Learn to open tab-topped drinks.
Find the apple on your button-talker.
Count to four by clapping hands (imitate).

Mr. Bob opened the ARD with the observation that Ben's receptive language—his understanding—had increased, and that he was following directions better. I was glad that Mr. Bob had noticed. In fact, I'd made sure of it. I'd gone to his classroom, handed Ben a wad of paper, and told him, "Throw it away." Ben had walked across the room to the wastebasket and dropped it in. Perfect. Then I gave Mr. Bob a list of commands that Ben had been trained to follow in therapy: pick up, fasten, push, put in. I asked him to help me generalize these commands to the classroom. Mr. Bob was impressed with Ben's blossoming abilities.

From my own childhood and experience as a pupil in elementary school, I believed that teachers knew how to teach, just as doctors knew how to heal. Only slowly and reluctantly did I surrender the belief that professionals knew what was best for my child. In Ben's case, they did not. My experience for the past three years had been that special educators knew little or nothing that could help recover Ben. They didn't even think he *could* be recovered.

Ben could learn. I was sure of that. As my conviction grew, my anger grew. Finally, I'd had enough: the rules, the jargon, the pretensions. I pulled out the two-page list of learning objectives that I'd attached to the last IEP, one year earlier. My hands shaking, I began reading down it and asking questions. Could Ben open tab-topped soft drinks? Could he find the apple button on his talker? Could he count to four by clapping his hands four times?

Mr. Bob said that these goals were reinforced throughout the school day. It was an honest answer, and he was a decent man, kind to the kids. But I was ready to vent my anger at this delusional system, and he was standing in the line of fire.

"So how successful is he at each of these tasks," I asked. "Fifty percent? Seventy percent? Has he mastered any of them?"

"Some," Mr. Bob answered.

"Which ones?"

"Well, the buttons. He's getting better at that."

"How much better? Where is the supporting data?" I asked.

Of course, there wasn't any.

"How about the next objective," I asked, "to count to four by clapping?" My hands were still shaking, but I was determined to go down the list item by item if necessary.

Ms. Upchurch, the principal, came to his rescue. "Mr. Burns," she said, "you pick Ben up every day at two o'clock for his home speech program. School isn't over until three o'clock." She reached into her jargon bag and pulled out a term fraught with legal implications. "We cannot be responsible for meeting your objectives with these *excessive absences.*"

I had a jargon bag of my own, and it had one item in it. A slingshot. I picked it up and loaded it with a term I'd learned at the Dallas Autism Society.

"According to law," I said, "Ben is entitled to a *free and appropriate education.* The education he is receiving here is not appropriate." And the proof of that was his abysmal three-year evaluation.

"What do you want, Mr. Burns?" demanded the principal.

I hadn't planned to say this, but I was emboldened by my anger. "I want the school district to pay for Ben's Lovaas program, forty hours a week," I said. "Starting last year."

"I'm declaring this a Disagreement ARD," said Ms. Upchurch. "This committee will recess."

❺   ❺   ❺

On May 28, 1996, the disagreement went to mediation. In attendance at the mediation session were Dr. Dorothy Bennett, the director of Special Education, and the Autism Queen.

"Dr. Burns, do you believe in recovery?" asked Dr. Bennett.

Of course I believed in recovery. I was convinced that Ben, like the children in the Lovaas study, had at least a chance of raising his IQ and becoming indistinguishable, socially and intellectually, from children who had never been autistic. But I had never discussed this conviction with his teachers or administrators. "Autistic children don't recover." That dogma, pervasive in the DISD school system, was like a heavy blanket, a snowfall, an avalanche, covering any hope of recovery, paralyzing the system, precluding discussion, bringing Ben's progress to a halt, stuck in the snow drifts.

Dr. Bennett was asking for a confession of my misguided faith so she could attack it. In truth, I found it difficult to confess. I wanted the school system to validate my belief. I wanted Ben's teachers to look at his progress and say, "This is astonishing. He's not the same child he was six months ago. I've never seen anything like it. Are you sure he's autistic? Maybe the doctors made a mistake." Instead, his teachers minimized his accomplishments.

"You're working on language at home two hours a day?" a teacher had said. "I see progress, but not two hours a day."

I had been waiting on the school system's permission to believe in Ben's recovery. Now I knew that permission would never come, but I didn't need it. I turned to Dr. Bennett and walked the plank. "Yes, I believe in recovery," I said. "Don't you?"

My question put Dr. Bennett on the spot. If she said yes, the next question was, "How many autistic children has your TEACCH program recovered?" If she answered no, why did she deserve to be Director of Special Education?

The Autism Queen jumped in. "You can't raise a child's IQ. Lovaas used only high-functioning children in his experiments. The results he claimed to have achieved have never been duplicated."

"The duplication studies are underway," I said. "Should we wait for further evidence, or take our best shot with Ben?"

In the end, I won. Or so I thought. Ben would be provided with a one-on-one aide who would be selected in consultation with me. The aide would be trained in "direct teaching techniques," which I assumed would be Lovaas therapy, by a consultant mutually accept-able to the school and me. The Autism Queen would rewrite Ben's IEP goals to make them measurable, and the school would collect data on Ben's progress, reported to me daily and weekly. Case con-ferences would be scheduled every six weeks.

The mediated agreement looked good on paper. I was satis-fied. Though it wasn't my original plan, I had been awarded an aide for Ben.

🐦   🐦   🐦

Sharon Hawkins, Ben's newly hired aide, was in a tight spot—between a rock and a hard place. The rock, her employer: a school system that didn't believe in recovery. The hard place: my insistence that Ben could learn to do anything we had the patience to teach him. Ben and I were early for our first meeting with her that June of 1996, at E. D. Walker. We made our way to Room 112, which was to be Ben's new homeroom, near the lavatory. Good. Eight-year-old Ben still had the occasional potty accident.

Room 112 was empty except for a few desks and some boxes stacked against the wall. Ben and I were alone under the fluorescent lights. I found a Barney puzzle, sat him down at a desk, and went to work. I took out Barney's head, offered it to Ben, guided his hand as he replaced it. Then Barney's feet and tail.

"Ben?" Speaking was a tall young African American woman with a kindly face. "Hi, I'm Sharon." She had a warm smile, and she had greeted Ben first. I liked her instantly. So far, I had not found anyone in the school system, except Ms. Seevers, who could teach Ben much of anything. Would Sharon be the exception? I walked her through a list of Ben's capabilities. I wanted her to focus on his strengths, not his deficits.

"Look, Ben can open the door," I said. "Open the door, Ben. See, he can open the door," I jabbered. "He can turn off lights, too." Was I really as nervous as I sounded? "Look, Ben, turn off the light. Good. Now turn it back on."

Ben turned on the light, walked over to the desk, picked up a puzzle piece, and dropped it on the floor.

"We've been working on this puzzle," I said to Sharon. "Maybe you could take over." I was trying to sound casual, but this was a test. She bent over to pick up the puzzle piece.

"No," I said, perhaps a little too harshly. "Make him pick it up."

Sharon took all the puzzle pieces out, put them on the desk in front of Ben, turned her back, and retreated. *This is not going to work*, I thought. But Sharon hadn't been trained yet. The school had promised to do that. I left Ben and Sharon alone.

Sharon's job, as she saw it, was to protect Ben from capricious demands, to fill in for his deficits, to be his mind, his feet, his hands. I saw her job as the opposite: to force him out of his comfort zone. In truth, Ben needed to be protected from a school system that was sometimes rigidly inflexible and from kids who could be cruel. And Sharon had one powerful quality that I lacked: patience. Her motto was, "If we don't get it today, we will get it tomorrow."

There were lots of tomorrows. Though I could not have known it at the time, Sharon was to stay with Ben as his aide and shadow for the next twelve years. In the early days, she protected him from his tantrums, from his own self-abusing anger. She called herself his mother at school, and sometimes she really did seem to stand in for Sue, keeping Ben clean, safe, fed, calm, and sheltered. He took his naps in her lap. She was family.

The school system had promised to hire a consultant in "direct teaching techniques" to train Sharon. I had to press them: repeated phone calls, lost messages, slow returns. Eventually my reminder made its way through the chaotic system, and Dr. Bennett offered a candidate: a clinical psychologist from Tulsa who made her living conferring with schools in Oklahoma and Texas. I requested the opportunity to meet the consultant and see her in action. Dr. Bennett seemed surprised. What action?

"I'd like to see her at work in the classroom."

Bennett, hamstrung by the mediation agreement, couldn't refuse.

        ❧   ❧   ❧

Mr. Bob kept a pleasant, orderly classroom. Sunlight flooded in though the large east windows. Jason was in the corner, sitting on his potty chair. Ben walked aimlessly around the room, picking up objects and putting them in his mouth. The consultant, old enough to have grown up dancing to the Beatles, was dressed in scarves, long earrings, and sandals, and was wearing enough perfume to alter global weather patterns. I mentally nicknamed her Ms. Windhover. She followed Ben in his aimless, repetitive pacing but had no interaction with him or with Sharon.

"What are you doing?" I asked her.

"I am evaluating the classroom environment and observing your son."

"What are your observations?" I asked. Was too much sunlight coming into the room? Were the pictures mounted too high or too low?

"I will report my observations to the school system," Ms. Windhover replied. "Now, is there anything else?"

"Yes, a teaching demonstration," I answered. "I would like to see you teach Ben something." The teaching staff, Sharon, Mr. Bob, and his assistants, were watching.

"What do you mean, teach him something?"

"How about following two-step instructions," I suggested. I pulled out the list of objectives that I had attached to his IEP. "Get a red crayon out of the supply box, and close the box."

"That's not fair," she said.

"Well, then, teach him to button his shirt."

"I am not a physical therapist, Mr. Burns."

"OK," I said. "You choose. Here is Ben's IEP." I handed her the list of instructional objectives.

No one rescued Ms. Windhover. She huffed out of the classroom, trailing perfume, and complained to the school system that I was being unreasonable and unfair. For the first time, I had the feeling that the teaching staff was on my side. They looked at me admiringly.

"Good work," said Sharon. Mr. Bob smiled and nodded in agreement.

❧   ❧   ❧

Judy Young, the next candidate, had worked for the Callier Center, the speech and hearing clinic at the University of Texas at Dallas. She'd been trained as a Lovaas therapist. And she had a sense of humor.

"What's Ben's favorite TV show?" she asked.

"*Wheel of Fortune*," I answered. "And *The Weather Channel*."

"Yep," she said. "Same as my other clients." She'd learned a lot from them. "If I'm assaulted in the parking lot, I know what to do."

"What?"

"Fall forward." Like Ben when he was resisting a lesson.

Judy had studied speech therapy in Europe and had a different approach. She explained that Ben was dyspraxic.

"What does that mean?" asked Sue.

"He has trouble sequencing the motor movements that he needs to make sounds," she explained. Ben would have to relearn how to talk, like a stroke victim. But speech was social, Judy believed, so she started with the social graces.

I gave a get-acquainted dinner. She taught Ben to scoot his chair up to the table.

Judy could get sounds out of Ben that no one else could get. She put her fingers in his mouth and moved his tongue. But sounds and words weren't her primary concern. She believed that the core communication skill was turn-taking. So she played games with Ben:

leapfrog, put the marble in the hole, anything that could be broken down into your turn/my turn. She gave him kinetic feedback: arm squeezes, belly rubs. She had him move his fingers one at a time, imitating her.

"He can learn to talk by moving his hands?" asked Sue.

"Externalizing the model makes it easier for him to observe, analyze, and imitate fine motor movements," she said. "Then we'll apply those skills to speech."

Judy observed that Ben liked weird things: plastic frog guts, mean-looking rubber dogs, scary books and pictures. She gave him choices: "Ben, do you want the monster ball or the frog guts?"

"Guts," said Ben.

I'd found an ally.

~   ~   ~

Nine months after Ben's three-year assessment, I requested a retest. It was scheduled for October 15, 1996, before Ben's annual late-October regression. By the retest, all systems were go. Ben had received five immunoglobulin infusions and was on a reduced-gluten, reduced-casein diet. His ear infections had abated. He'd also had nine months of additional discrete trial therapy and allergy shots. He was a different child than he had been nine months earlier: calm, focused, engaged.

In the antechamber, while I sipped my coffee from a Styrofoam cup, Ben picked up a toy truck and pushed it along the play rug road, unprompted.

"Mr. Burns," Ms. Varley said, "I'm ready for Ben." Ben and I walked in to the testing room together. Two hours later we walked out, and shortly thereafter I received her report.

"Compared to the assessment session completed in January 1996," she wrote, "Benjamin appeared physically healthier and less distressed and distractible. He has improved in his ability to attend to tasks and to tolerate direct instruction. He responded well to prompts to greet and say goodbye to people … he was able to verbalize and name some objects with one-word approximations."

Bottom line: in nine months, Ben's ceiling scores had increased from forty-one months to sixty months, a gain of nineteen months. Best of all, his mental age had increased from twenty-four months to thirty-seven months, a gain of thirteen months over a nine-month period. In short, Ben was gaining 1.4 months of mental age for every month of therapy. I thought this was a tremendous accomplishment, a fantastic pace. At that rate, by his mid-twenties, Ben's mental age would equal his chronological age. We were on a roll. And I was sure that with Judy's continued help, and with Sue and me on the same page, we could ramp up the program to reach that goal much faster.

COLD WAR

Joining forces for Ben, Sue and I looked for a place to settle in together. During the spring of 1997, I drew circles and lines on the map—school, Bachman Recreation Center, routes to work. All pointers intersected at a block of older apartments just a short hike from Gooch Elementary, Ben's school. The once-proud apartments, gone to seed and drug dealers, were being gutted and renovated, like me. Southern-mansion style, low-rise, verandas, hanging gardens, over-sized rooms, lavish space; real plaster on the foot-thick walls, steel and brick superstructure built to last a century. Bay windows looking out on the oak-shaded lawn. Playground and a swimming pool just around the corner. Foliage at the bottom of the stairs where Sue could plant a garden.

We rented a three-bedroom apartment on the second floor: master for Sue, study/bedroom for me, cubby for Ben. My Mom and Dad bought us a new washer and dryer set, blessing our reunion. The dining room table doubled as Ben's therapy desk, where trainers could sit. Searching the Salvation Army for treasures, I selected a Queen Anne sofa and matching chair recovered in green fleur-de-lis. I paid from my savings and offered it as a gift to Sue, an open hope chest. She branded the living room with a red fleur-de-lis mismatched chair. Her mark.

Sue and I had joined more than our physical living quarters; we had picked up the pieces from Ben's freefall and merged our expectations. Ben had a single home with consistent rules. His smile returned, lighting up the apartment, warming our hearts. Ben was back. So was Sue. And moonflowers sprang up among the foliage at the foot of the stairs that fall.

By November of 1997, the pieces of ten-year-old Ben's recovery program were in place. As I anticipated, Ben benefited from consistent rules in the new household, though sometimes not without prodding.

"Ben, wipe the table," Sue commanded, yelling at him from the kitchen. He did nothing.

"Wipe it!" she yelled, louder. Nothing.

Discipline and consistent rules entail not just what to require, but how to teach the requirement. So I broke the task down into steps. Get a sponge, turn on the water, wet the sponge. Divide the table into sections, wipe each section. I went over each step with Ben, hand over hand, while Sue watched. Soon she was using this step-by-step methodology to teach Ben to sweep the floor and brush his teeth.

Ben was also making great progress in language. He received the Most Improved Student Award as school. When I turned off the TV, he said, "Stop that, Dad." A day or two later we had our first real discussion.

"Pear," he said, picking up a yellow apple.

"No, Ben, that's an apple," I explained.

"Pear," he insisted.

I wrote a book, "Pat the Pup," using only words that Ben could read or at least say. Sue illustrated it. Ben's teachers read it to him at school, and he said the words right along with them. Watching a video at school, Ben said "pup" when a picture of a dog came on the screen. He identified other animals: "Cat. Bird." He was proud of himself, showing off his verbal skills. Instead of pushing his teachers' hands toward objects he wanted, he used a new phrase to make requests. It sounded like "wanta" or "wattha." Mr. Bob thought he was asking for water and took him to the water fountain to get drinks. "He drank water all day," he told me. We laughed about that when I explained that "wanta" meant *want that*, an all-purpose request.

I had never been more optimistic about his prospects. The school system had committed significant resources. Judy Young was working directly with Ben and training and supervising Sharon. One of Mr. Bob's assistants, Miss Dee, a talented teacher, had a special interest in Ben and worked with him during school hours. I had a rotation team of trainers coming to the apartment five days a week for drills. Even Deborah, our neighbor, a qualified teacher who had recently lost her son to AIDS, volunteered to work with me and the school system to integrate games with the drills and make learning fun for Ben. I sensed—and the teachers agreed—that Ben was on the verge of a breakthrough in language. "He's *ready*," said Miss Dee. But there was another time bomb waiting to explode.

❧   ❧   ❧

By late March 1998, when I went into Ben's room to help him get dressed, change a video, or kiss him goodnight, he crawled into my lap, gave me hugs, sometimes seized me and held on for minutes. In the mirror, I could see Sue hovering around the doorway, keeping an eye on us. "I'll bet she thinks I'm sexually abusing Ben," I thought. I should have addressed the issue, but I ignored it. "She'll get over it," I said to myself.

Midnight, early April 1998. Ten-year-old Ben couldn't sleep. So Sue couldn't sleep. Fragmented memories of her father's repeated threats and rapes washed over her like waves. I gave Ben three milligrams of melatonin, a natural hormone that resets the sleep-wake cycle, but it wouldn't take effect for an hour. Might was well use the time doing language drills. Putting my hands on Ben's shoulders, I guided him to the therapy table.

"Get your hands off Ben." It was the White Bitch.

She was standing, bathrobed, in the doorway to her bedroom. Rage swelled up in me. I said the most hurtful thing that came to mind, a line that could have been written by the director of Auschwitz, or by Sue's dad:

"You worthless fucking bitch."

Instant gratification. Sue barricaded herself in her bedroom.

When my anger abated, I recognized that, in her mind, she was merely defending her son. I'd have done the same. The next day, I wrote her a note: "I'm glad you are my partner in recovering Ben."

She dropped the note on the floor, a distant look on her face.

We went on with our lives, but I feared that Sue would exercise her own version of the Golden Rule: "Do unto others whatsoever they do unto you." She remained polite on the surface, but she was seething with anger beneath. When the three of us went on a city-sponsored run, she pushed ahead, turned off the marked path, left Ben and me in the dust. The tectonic plates were shifting again. When would the next earthquake occur?

It was the last Saturday in May of 1998. Sue planned an overnight family trip to Lake Murray, a state park, our traditional getaway spot in southern Oklahoma, between Dallas and Stillwater. Sue wanted to go in two cars, but I planned to sit in the back seat of my Honda to teach Ben prepositions while Sue drove. The car was a great venue for language drills because Ben couldn't run away from his lesson. Sue resisted the single-car strategy, but didn't give a reason. I missed the cue.

That night, Ben slept between Sue and me. He snuggled up to me. I woke up feeling that Ben and I were being watched. Sue had pulled the sheet off of us. She was sitting up, staring at us as she had done back in the apartment. I covered up and went back to sleep.

The next morning Sue sent Ben and me to the lodge for breakfast but stayed in the cabin by herself. When I got back, she had packed up. "I want you to take Ben and me home," she said. "Then get out of the apartment. I can't live with a child abuser."

I was stunned. "What are you talking about?"

"I saw you last night, half awake, your hands all over Ben. You would have raped him if I hadn't stopped you."

Her accusation hit me between the eyes. Like many gay men, I was plagued by internalized homophobia on the issue of pedophilia. Then the bad news came out. While Ben and I were at breakfast, she'd called the police, and they had alerted Child Protective Services (CPS) in Dallas.

Back in Dallas that afternoon, Sue moved out, taking Ben with her. And I received a call from a CPS staffer. She wanted to interview Ben.

"You're making a big mistake," I said. "His mother is delusional. And she's not my wife. I can explain everything."

"I can see you at three o'clock, for ten minutes."

I arrived on time to the appointment. Who was this person? I glanced around the office for clues. Behind her desk was a diploma, prominently displayed, of her associate's degree from Ambassador College, Church of God. "We Stand for the King." She had just graduated.

The staffer got right to the point. "Mr. Burns, did you ever appear unclothed in front of your son or your other children?"

"Yes, of course." The swimming pool, the men's dressing room.

"That is all I need to know. I'll escort you to the door."

"What do you mean, that's all you need to know?"

"You exposed yourself to a minor. That is child abuse in Texas. You are a self-confessed child abuser, Mr. Burns. I will issue a protective order for Ben and file charges on his behalf with the district attorney."

🐌　　🐌　　🐌

As a gay man, I suspected that I would be presumed guilty until proven innocent. Jack Hampton, a prominent Dallas district court judge, had stated from the bench that he considered gays on the same level as prostitutes.

I hired an attorney, a specialist in family law.

"The first thing I'll do," promised the lawyer, "is quash the CPS staffer."

I wasn't sure what quashing meant, but it sounded like something I would personally like to do with a large rock.

"Yes, quash her." I wrote the attorney a check for the last $1,200 in my savings account.

Eventually, the district attorney dropped the charges against me, but the battle over Ben dragged on. I sued for custody. Sue countersued. Legal bills mounted and threatened to bankrupt us both. Eventually Sue called me at work to propose a deal. "Let's just go back to the old system," she said. I agreed. It was better than the precipice toward which we were stumbling. We would continue to live separately, and Ben would split his days and nights between us.

I surveyed the damage. On the plus side, much of Ben's recovery system was still intact. Judy Young, Ben's speech therapist, continued to see him. He still had Sharon and his support system at school. I'd found a pharmacy in the Rio Grande Valley that would compound transdermal secretin, a natural hormone that had a dramatic effect on some autistic kids, and Ben improved on that treatment for a while.

But my heart wasn't in Ben's program. The momentum I'd worked so hard to build was lost. I felt that the teachable moment had passed, Candlestick Park swallowed by a sinkhole. The tag team of trainers drifted away. "Why don't you make up little songs and sing them to Ben anymore?" asked Sue. I didn't know I'd stopped singing.

Truth is, I was still in shock from Sue's charges. How could she have done that? In the end, what difference did my efforts make? Dr. Hitzfelder had been right. Ben was damaged beyond repair and would never fully recover.

From time to time a friend would call to share a new autism therapy from a TV program or a magazine article. I listened politely, tried to keep my antenna up, but the therapies were only new to the caller: allergy shots, secretin, diets, gamma globulin, prayer and energy fields, B6, DMG, and the dozens of dietary supplements and medical interventions reviewed in Dr. Rimland's *ARRI Newsletter*. Sue and I knew them all. We had opened every door and walked down every path.

AFTERSHOCKS

Within a few months, Sue's apartment deteriorated, the second one she'd trashed. Roaches erupted and multiplied as if by spontaneous generation, hatched from festering food. The apartment smelled like a cat box. Judy refused to do therapy at Sue's. She brought Ben over to my apartment. "Sue said something about my mother that was so repulsive and hurtful that I can't repeat it."

"Oh, that wasn't really Sue," I explained, "That was the White Bitch."

"I'm not going back there."

Sue didn't see her apartment as a rattrap; she saw it as a treasure box. She'd dubbed herself the Salvage Queen of Dallas. When an old Highland Park mansion was scheduled for demolition, she'd sneak into the site looking for collectibles, pull up in her red Ford Escort, branded with yellow-and-green sunflowers the size of basketballs painted on the car. Camouflage, she thought, but it stood out like a circus clown car. She packratted chandeliers, fancy light switches, window boxes, exotic plants, carpets, drapes, and once even ten pounds of wild rice, found in the upper reaches of an abandoned pantry. She made art, kinetic sculptures, wind chimes, hanging mobiles, vases, and planters out of these recovered treasures, and she populated her living quarters with them.

Ben had trouble sleeping through the nights at Sue's. He'd climb to the second floor and run up and down the outside hallway, opening neighbors' doors, run on the edge of the roof toward the full moon. I put a deadbolt on the inside of Sue's door, higher than Ben could reach at the time, but it didn't work for long. Sue gave eleven-year-old Ben human growth hormone—God knows where and why she got it—and he went through puberty early, shot up like a weed.

I'd have rescued Ben from that environment, and probably should have tried, but Sue had proved that she held the high card. All she had to do was call CPS and allege sexual abuse. "Gay Dad," I imagined my file was titled. They'd issue another thirty-day protective order, pull Ben from school, escort him to the hospital, and check for anal penetration as they had before. Nothing would be found, but Ben would suffer invasion, shame and embarrassment.

Up until the confrontation with CPS, my recovery work with Ben followed a pattern. Driven to the edge of my limitations and fears, I took a step into the unknown, found my footing. This time I didn't take the step. Sue had me over a barrel. I was afraid of losing Ben.

🙠   🙠   🙠

On the Fourth of July, 2000, about midnight, I answered a knock on the door. The apartment manager was silhouetted against an orange sky.

"Fire!"

Flames leapt from the apartments half a block to the west, where twelve-year-old Ben was staying with Sue. I grabbed my billfold and cell phone and ran to the street, found Sue and Ben among the milling crowd.

"Come on guys," said Sue to the firefighters. "Hook it up. That's right. Now turn it on. Good job. Now aim it at my apartment." They were too slow for her. "I'm going back in," Sue shouted. Fire raged through the common attic space. Sue came out with a portfolio of watercolors.

Sue camped out on my front porch that night, watching the dying glow of the conflagration that destroyed her apartment, her treasure box, and the balanced life we had built around Ben.

By next morning, the TV crews had set up their mobile stations. Sue dragged out a large, soggy, smoked painting and gave an interview. Ben and I rode our bikes to the safety barricades that surrounded the wreckage. He'd stare, cycle back to my apartment, then return to the barricades behind Sue's for more staring.

"It burned, Ben. Big fire," I said. "But you're OK. Mommy's OK."

That afternoon Sue asked me to help with the salvage operation. The courtyard and walkways were flooded, the apartment damaged by heat, smoke, and water. She wanted to retrieve Ben's bed.

"Sue, the barricades are there for a reason," I argued.

I'd seen her in situations like this before. Her strategy, when faced with a barrier, was to plunge ahead, beyond her abilities and limits, expecting someone to rescue her. I'd visited her in the hospital when she'd tried to lift a piano using a stick as a lever. No one stepped in to help. The piano fell on her foot.

"If you won't help," said Sue outside her ruined apartment, "I'll do it myself."

We backpacked out black garbage bags of Ben's clothes, water-soaked socks, paintings, jewelry, tools, dishes. Ben's antique brass bed. Wading through the water-filled courtyard, Sue fell into a hole, stuck. I pulled her out.

Back at my apartment, Sue was fixing up her old bathroom, which had fallen into disrepair. She scrubbed out the mold, reattached the toilet seat, and wanted to remount the shower curtain. I didn't know it at the time, but she was trying to make a decision: to stay, or not to stay. She asked me to go to Home Depot and pick up a wooden dowel. I bought an adjustable curtain rod instead. Sue was furious. The argument escalated.

"You didn't want to help me move my stuff out."

"I pulled you out of a hole. Rescued you, as usual."

Angry, Sue drove her flowermobile north on Marsh Lane for several miles until she found an apartment complex with a "For Rent" sign. It was off the path, out of the way, but it had a weight room and a pool. She rented it on the spot.

The fight hadn't been about the materials. The fight had been about our relationship. "I wanted to know," said Sue, "if there was a place for me."

After she left, I went through the abandoned master bedroom. The yellow legal-pad note was still in the corner, where Sue had dropped it years ago.

I read what I had written: "I'm glad you are my partner in recovering Ben." I threw the note in the wastebasket. Dr. Kotsanis had retired. Bill McKnight had accepted a position in another city. I had stopped demanding the data sheets on Ben's language drills that the school was supposed to be sending weekly—blood from a stone— and the school had stopped sending them.

Six years after it had begun, The Benjamin Project was over.

PART 4

NEVER GIVE UP

Over the Rainbow

In August of 2001, the summer that Ben turned fourteen, I bought a condominium in Oak Lawn, a leafy, gentrified Dallas enclave near the city center. Sue would pick Ben up from school, feed him her home-cooked gluten-free dinners, and bring him to me for the night. We alternated weekends for a while, but Ben slept better at my place. He stayed. Ben and I became a family unit. Letters arrived in my mailbox addressed to "Dan and Ben."

I poured myself into my work and taught an overload: as many as seventeen sections of communications courses, mostly online. In the evenings, Ben watched TV or read Dr. Seuss books while I e-mailed my students and graded papers, listening to WRR, the Dallas classical station. Tchaikovsky piano concertos, Mozart, or Bach played in the background. About nine thirty, I'd wind up the evening.

"Ben, do you want to go to Lucky's?"

He'd nod yes, and we were off for bedtime snacks, steamed broccoli, or red beans and rice, at the corner café, floor-to-ceiling windows looking out over pedestrian traffic and the upscale urban landscape.

Lucky's was a great place for people watching—artists, couples, panhandlers, professionals. But I watched Ben. As he looked out the window or at the TV, his face reflected a rich internal life: shades of emotion ever shifting, variable as the shadow of leaves in a summer breeze. Concentration, affirmation, curiosity, surprise, delight. A happy couple, we ate our snacks and drank our wine and lemonade in companionable silence.

Friday afternoons I'd pick Ben up from school early and haul the bikes to Cedar Creek State Park, the best mountain bike trail in North Texas, or to Oak Cliff Nature Preserve, Lake Ray Roberts, the Katy Trail, or Boulder Park. On the mountain bike trails, Ben didn't seem autistic. He rode the bike exactly as I did; we were subject to the same laws of gravity. Long summer evenings, when I wasn't teaching, we cycled the Katy Trail, an old, abandoned railroad track turned into a scenic bike trail system that runs through Reverchon Park and uptown Dallas. After a great ride, hugs.

So passed the weekends, the years.

Late one summer, just before Ben turned sixteen, we coasted our bikes toward the Boulder Park dam, down the asphalt driveway parallel to a dense cedar forest laced by looping trails.

"On every turn," the guidebook warned, "one will inevitably encounter a new trail that appears from nowhere. Refer to map." But the map looked to me like the trace of sparklers swung by kids on the Fourth of July, loops within loops. I knew that the main trails crossed at right angles on the high ground near two piles of asphalt pointing toward the creek. From there I could find my way back to the dam.

I took a sip of bottled water and checked my watch. Plenty of daylight left, I thought, though a shadow flickered across my mind as I recalled that July days were getting shorter. I made a mental note of the time: 7:10 p.m. Ben had circled back to see what was holding me up. The trail was moist with a carpet of cedar fallings that showed fresh tire tracks. Normally Ben and I were the only people in this wilderness park, and that was the way I liked it. I rode behind him, as usual, so I could keep an eye on him. I shoved the water bottle deep into my pocket.

"Ben, turn right," I shouted, and followed him down the unknown trail and into the darkening woods.

By 7:20 we had come to the creek crossing. The upper fork of the trail swerved up an embankment, over a four-foot concrete pipe, then back to the other side. Ben tried to take the lower fork, which ran through the water, but I called out to him and led us up the slope. From there the trail veered toward a darker part of the forest. "The Tulgey Wood," I thought, with branches that reached down to scrape and grab. Ben whipped by them, ducking, his bike weaving, and I followed.

By 7:30 the woods were noticeably darker. Time to head home. Looking for familiar territory, I decided to follow a deeply rutted trail west, toward Boulder Drive. The moon was straight ahead of us. *It rises in the west, doesn't it?* I noticed bicycle tracks on the path. Been, here, I thought. Good. But had we? I saw heaps of old shingles and asphalt, but not the twin mounds.

When we came to the creek, it was flowing the wrong direction. Ben and I scurried down the steep, muddy bank, splashed through the water, and scrambled our way up the other side. No matter how I tried to mentally twist and turn the landscape, it didn't fit any known pattern. We were lost. But even in the darkening woods, I knew up from down. "Up, Ben!" I yelled.

He rode ahead of me, disappearing into the dark.

"Ben, stay with me!" I shouted.

"Guhg" he yelled back. Then I caught sight of him. Nothing on the high ground looked familiar until Ben stopped at a point where the trails crossed. He'd found the twin mounds.

If there was a single, dramatic turning point from grief to acceptance, it occurred when Ben and I, biking, rose over the ridge at Cedar Hill State Park, the lake shimmering below. Ben was wearing his "Reclaiming the Mind" T-shirt, and as I saw him silhouetted against the lake and sky, I felt my spirit soar. I lived in the afterglow of that moment for weeks. A song we sang in church brought it back:

And the heavens open when you speak to me
Pouring light into my waiting heart,
And the music fills an ocean silently, quietly,
When you speak to me.

Ben was silent, but Abba spoke to me through my love for my son. I hadn't given up hope for Ben. Yet for me, for now, Ben was not a problem to be solved but a song to be sung.

ș   ș   ș

As Ben grew into his teen years, his grandmother stepped in to fill the gap. Grandma Jeanne visited his school events, Halloween parties, Special Olympics. She bought him clothes and toys. She paid for his horseback-riding lessons and encouraged him. "He's our Benjamin," she told me.

We took him every August, his birthday month, to the Sears portrait store at Redbird Mall for an annual portrait. The series of photographs show an alert boy blossoming into a handsome young teen.

At age fifteen, the photograph shows a sensitive boy with intense eyes. "A young James Dean," as Sharon said.

"You're a big boy now, Ben," said Sue. "You're going to high school. Do you want to go to high school?"

Ben nodded yes, but he looked like somebody facing his first skydive. On August 26, 2002, with Sharon in support, Ben was to join the prevocational class at W. T. White High School in Dallas.

Sue and I parked at the church across the playing field from the school and walked him over. We congratulated each other. With Sharon's help, we hoped, Ben would hold a job in the work-study program, gain knowledge from his teachers, and learn from his peers.

Ben's first day on the job, I snuck into Wal-Mart with my camera, crept through the labyrinth of aisles. If Ben saw a camera pointed at him, he would turn toward it and open his mouth, waiting for the flash. Sharon knew I was coming.

I spotted them in the women's accessories department, putting colorful summer clothes on hanging racks. I signaled to Sharon and snuck around behind the rack of nightgowns. She put a garment in his hand, pointed to an empty hanger, and said, "Put on." Then she guided his hand to make sure the nightgown was positioned correctly. I got off one flash. Ben saw me with the camera and mugged. He was so proud of himself. And I was so proud of my son.

At age sixteen, Ben's annual Sears portrait shows a tanned, healthy-looking teen with a direct gaze and a hint of a smile. That year, at Luby's cafeteria, Ben's job was to put the sugar packets in the white plastic sugar caddies. Sharon would seat him at a table, arrange the sugar caddy and the box of sugar packets in front of him, point, and say, "Put in." He was practicing his matching skills. Sharon would check his work to make sure that the packets were all facing the same way.

At age seventeen, the annual portrait shows his usual good-humored face and his large tan hands grasping a football. That year, Ben worked at Cici's Pizza, the high school student store, and the high school cafeteria. Sharon would organize and manage the work, and Ben would do it. I thought about how it wasn't that different from the system where I worked at University of Texas Arlington, supervising programmers on a U.S. Defense Department contract. I organized the work, prioritized the tasks, communicated with management. The workers wrote the code. Though Ben's tasks were much simpler, he was learning the basic work model from the ground up.

In June 2005, Sharon summed up her nine-year relationship with seventeen-year-old Ben. She had these words printed and framed:

Ben only lets a few people into his world. I was blessed to be one of those he let in. He has taught me that it is OK to be different and that it is OK to keep trying to understand. Most importantly, he has taught me to live and to love and for that reason, he is precious and special to me.

At age eighteen, in the annual portrait, Ben's smile had parted to show teeth. He appears to be a confident, laughing youngster. But good spirits masked a growing problem. That year, Charlotte Barber had taken over Ben's prevocational class and raised the average test scores by instilling order and discipline. Her classroom was a mixed blessing for Ben. Though he benefited from some of the more structured activities, he had a difficult time attending to the more scholarly lessons and the increased focus on testing and academics.

Near the end of the school year, tests behind them, teachers and students were relaxing a bit and letting off steam. When I visited the classroom, Ben was sitting at his desk waving some coat hangers over his head.

"Put them down," said Ms. Barber.

Ben threw the coat hangers onto the floor and jammed his fingers into his ears. He seemed to enjoy provoking the teacher.

"Pick them up, Ben," said Ms. Barber.

Ben jammed his fingers deeper into his ears.

"I'm getting out my yardstick," said Ms. Barber. She was playing with him. "It's been a long time since I've used my yardstick." She waved it in the air like a Star Wars laser sword.

Ben closed his eyes and slumped deeper into the desk, shutting out the world. WHACK. Ms. Barber slapped his desk with her yardstick. Ben opened his eyes and looked up at her.

"Pretty!" he said.

"Are you flirting with me, Ben?" asked Ms. Barber.

Ben smiled. "Yes."

By age nineteen, the Special Ed class had advanced two grade levels since Ms. Barber took over. But Ben wasn't keeping up, and his hyperacusis—his painfully sensitive hearing—was worse. He was plugging his ears almost constantly. At school, seated away from the other students, head down, eyes closed, fingers stuffed into his ears, Ben looked like the three wise monkeys—hear, speak, see no evil—rolled into one. When the air conditioning system roared like a Boeing 747, when the lunchroom rumbled like a cattle stampede, when the tardy bell clanged like a four-alarm fire, Ben would hunker down at his desk with his fingers in his ears and keep them there, sometimes all day.

"Give him time," I told the teacher. Time didn't help. Lulled into complacency, I failed to see that Ben's hyperacusis was steadily getting worse.

The last photograph in the series was taken not at the Sears studio but at Grace Presbyterian Village, where Mom had gone to spend her final days. As Ben waxed, she waned. But even there, she cared for Ben. When he had been up for two nights with an earache, she set him up comfortably in the dayroom at her rest home, wrapped him in an angel blanket, and sang to him until he fell asleep, his head on her shoulder.

With Mom's passing, it was time for a change.

※   ※   ※

In January 2006, bicycling the scenic Katy Trail, I imagined that Sue and I would have a magical child whom we would raise together. Swept along by a tide-like force, I felt that I was being lifted, like *E.T.'s* Elliott, toward the sky.

Sue had progressed in her therapy—she'd been at it for fifteen years—and had remarried. She'd been elected president of her Rotary Club. She was still, however, very angry. Her therapist said the anger was a dam for grief.

"I can't cry," Sue told me. "Dr. Dunckley said if I could cry, I could get well."

A few weeks later, around Sue's birthday, I was contemplating a black-and-white picture of her I'd taken shortly after we were married. I'd hung it over my desk.

The phone rang. It was Sue. "I've got to talk to you."

I looked at the photo. It showed her in a sailor suit, blonde hair in her eyes, Hang-on-Sloopy style, face turned up against the sun, the Sue I loved.

"I just saw a movie about recovered autistic children," Sue continued.

I sat up straight. Was this the call I'd been waiting for?

When Ben was fourteen, I'd read a paper authored by parents of autistic children: "Autism: A Novel Form of Mercury Poisoning," by Sallie Bernard and other parents and clinicians. I sensed that I was witnessing a milestone in medical history, like Louis Pasteur proposing germ theory. If we knew the "etiology" of autism, its cause, I was sure that effective medical treatments would follow.

And they had. By 2003, Dr. Rimland's Defeat Autism Now! (DAN!) organization, a consortium of doctors, parents, and scientists, was receiving a tide of reports of children recovering from autism. Hundreds of preschool kids, following the DAN! protocols, were shedding the Autism Spectrum Disorder diagnosis and going to first grade as if they had never been autistic. At the 2004 DAN! Conference, Dr. Rimland and his staff had invited a dozen of recovered kids on stage to be interviewed by a celebrity. That was the movie Sue had seen.

"All those years," said Sue, "when you talked about recovering Ben, I thought it was bullshit." She was furious.

"What do you think now?" I asked.

"Why isn't Ben up on that stage?"

That fall, Sue's Rotary Club was considering funding some cooking equipment and bus trips for Ben's class. I drove Ms. Barber to a noon luncheon to appeal to the Rotarians for their support. I was proud of my ex-wife, her position, her executive abilities.

"I want to thank Ms. Barber," said Sue, introducing the speaker, "for all she has done for …"

Sue's voice caught. She swayed at the podium as if she had been hit in the stomach, struggled for control.

"… all she has done for …"

She seemed so small, curled up, struggling to take a breath. In the fifteen years since Ben's diagnosis, I had seen Sue storming with rage, but I had never seen her shed a tear. She gritted her teeth, took a breath, and finished, tears streaming.

" … for my son."

The dam had burst.

Driven by Sue's flood of energy, we bought the videodiscs for the most recent DAN! Conference presentations—about twenty hours' worth of medical information—and took turns watching them, comparing notes and ideas.

"Did you see the Martha Herbert video about brain inflammation?" asked Sue.

"Yes. Maybe that's why Ben has a big head," I replied. "Did you see Jon Pangborn talking about methylation?"

Sue's excitement rekindled my own. I ordered Pangborn and Baker's *Autism: Effective Biomedical Treatments* and began searching for a DAN! doctor who could guide us through the complicated protocols.

I typed Dr. Kotsanis's name into Google. Up popped his current address and telephone number. Yes, Dr. Kotsanis remembered Ben well, and would be happy to see him again.

We arrived for our appointment on September 18, 2006. Following the doctor's advice, Sue and I tightened Ben's gluten-free diet and reduced his casein intake. When I put on my gluten- and casein-detecting goggles, most food products glowed orange: cookies, crackers, cake, breads, buns, malt, pasta, sodas, pizza, and about 25,000 brand- name products. They were Ben's favorite food, drinks, and treats, heavily advertised, prominently featured and on every menu, food shelf, refrigerator, and vending machine, within easy reach. I felt that I should have the right as a free American to purchase anything on a grocery store shelf without reading the fine print. But in reality Ben's health and safety were up to Sue and me. From time to time we were tempted to allow him gluten- and casein-free vacations, but Ben's leaky gut never went on vacation. Detoxing his diet became easier over time.

Dr. Kotsanis also prescribed glutathione and methyl-B12 shots. After Ben's metabolism regained its balance and his gut began to heal, he pronounced him ready for the next crucial step.

We began Ben's chelation, his detoxification, in December 2006: DMSA, or dimercaptosuccinic acid, three days on and four days off. Every three months, we measured Ben's progress with a challenge test, the Toxic Element Profile. "So we'll know," Dr. Kotsanis explained, "when to stop." The challenge test didn't show how much mercury and other heavy, toxic metals were left in Ben's body—there was no test for that—it showed how much was coming out.

Because the mercury, lead, and other toxins are deeply imbedded in body tissues, including brain cells, sometimes it takes a year or more to reduce the heavy metals and other toxins to "undetectable levels," too little to show up on the challenges.

For the first three months, lead came pouring out. "I was tearing down a lead-painted barn when I was pregnant," said Sue. "I'd forgotten about that."

Six months into the protocol, Ben began excreting significant quantities of mercury. "We've got the culprit," said Dr. Kotsanis. "We're shaking it loose." Ben took a five-week series of forty high-pressure hyperbaric oxygen treatments, supporting his detoxification, and we bought a home low-pressure hyperbaric chamber for home use. Finally, on my birthday, December 7, 2007, one year after we had begun, the doctor recommended that we cease chelation and move on to the next protocol.

More tests had revealed another problem, Pediatric Autoimmune Neuropsychiatric Disorder Associated with Streptococcus (PANDAS), a disease that attacks the basil ganglia, the communication channel between the lower and higher brain. "That could be why he's not talking," said Dr. Kotsanis. "It may also be driving his hyperacusis." He put Ben on a protocol of antibiotics, antivirals, and antifungals, plus probiotics to replace the good gut flora. Ben's symptoms improved. A follow-up PANDAS test showed seven out of twelve panels trending down. The doctor prescribed a mineral solution, chlorine dioxide. "It kills everything but the patient," he joked. But would it cure Ben's hyperacusis?

❧   ❧   ❧

Every summer, in Oklahoma at Burns Land, where Dorothy and Mary had lived, Pete gave a party. It was an echo of Dorothy and Mary's annual solstice party, but shifted to the Fourth of July weekend, traditionally a big holiday in the Burns family. On July 3, 2008, Sue and I filled my car trunk with bottled water and soft drinks, quite a load for a little old Honda Civic, and made the two-hundred-and-fifty mile drive, drilling Ben on language. Pete's friend Bruce, the fire master, came down from Pennsylvania to help roast a pig.

We were sitting around the pond, Pete and Troy drinking beer, Bruce cutting firewood with the chainsaw, Ben just sitting, when my cell phone rang. "This is Heather," said a young voice.

"He-Thor?" I asked. I wasn't hearing well. "What are you doing with Hannah's phone?"

"I found it."

"Where are you?" I asked.

"At Panini bread."

"Banana bread?"

Over the roar of the chainsaw I heard a guffaw and looked up. Pete and Troy were barely able to contain their laughter. I looked at Ben. He was laughing too. And his fingers were not in his ears.

"It's the best vacation I've ever had," Sue said as we pulled into her driveway. With Ben on the mend, I had to agree.

As he blew out his twenty-first birthday candles that August, we had something extra to celebrate. His hyperacusis had vanished.

GOING HOME

In September, Ben and I marched in the 2008 Alan Ross Texas Freedom Gay Pride Parade with our church, Cathedral of Hope. Marchers wore red, blue, green, or yellow shirts, rainbow colors, and the church's theme, A Rainbow People, reminded me of *The Wizard of Oz*.

As Ben and I waited for the parade to start, standing in the shade of a huge old cottonwood tree and sharing a blue snow cone, I thought about how far we had come, and not come. Two decades earlier we began our journey. Me, the Cowardly Lion, kicking holes in the wall and fearful that I was not up to the task of raising a disabled child. Sue, our Tin Man, rusty with grief. Ben, our Scarecrow with a head full of straw. The Yellow Brick Road is an image of the changes taking place in our lives, our journey, the gifts we have received.

Ben is a work in progress. The full force and fury of the autism storm have passed. Like New Orleans after Hurricane Katrina, damage is extensive and repair work is underway.

Standing there in the shade, sipping my melting blue snow cone, I made a mental list of Ben's recovery milestones. He hadn't had an ear infection since June of 2007. He slept through the night. He'd work a puzzle without prompting or redirecting until he finished it.

After dinner, he'd spend time with Sue and me in the living room, watching TV, reading, or just being part of the family. Ben would make direct, sustained, steady eye contact when I spoke to him. He read my facial expressions and used his own face to ask questions like "You want me to do what?" On our bike rides, he obeyed the commands "Stop!" and "Wait!" He made choices. He was patient. He was beginning to use a few words: *up, please, yes, no.* He could feed himself, go to the bathroom himself, and dress himself with supervision. He knew his left shoe from his right shoe. He picked up food crumbs took his empty plate to the kitchen. He brushed his teeth and washed his hair.

Much effort, modest results. Ben had not recovered. What if Sue and I had followed Dr. Hitzfelder's advice and saved our money for his institutionalization? Would we be richer? Would Ben be better off?

There were many roads I could have traveled. I could have nurtured my academic career, or followed my dream to write and produce a feature film. I could have volunteered for more mission trips for my church, perhaps traveled to those faraway places whose names entranced me from children's songs: Timbuktu, Constantinople, Tripoli. I could have followed my UTA lab boss to Washington, D.C., and perhaps made a much larger salary as a software engineer.

But there are many kinds of riches, and Ben touched me in a place that cannot be untouched. I cannot undo my love for him. Difficult as it was, I chose the right path for me and Ben. Into my third score of years, I am rich in experience, satisfaction, possibilities. I am no longer a human doing, but a human being. I have learned that you can lose everything except what you give away. That done, there is little left to fear.

What of Ben, his future? Where is the stage for children who don't fully recover and for adults for whom the biomedical revolution came late?

The parade began, and the crowd came alive with cheers and applause. Ben grinned and held his head high while I snapped a photo. He thought they were cheering for him. In a sense they were. The Alan Ross Texas Freedom Parade is not just about gay pride. It is about people who are different recognizing and celebrating their differences. It is about being yourself.

In *The Wizard of Oz*, the characters return from their Technicolor rainbow world to the black-and-white world of Kansas. But at the end of the movie there is something of the dream still clinging to Dorothy. She sees her home, her life, with new eyes. Weeks after the parade, I look at the photo I snapped of Ben. He is marching in front of three towering crosses, red, blue, and green, inscribed with *Paz, Liberación, Esperanza*. Peace, Liberation, and above all, Hope.

Though I look forward to more medical breakthroughs, I have learned that hope is not just a new protocol or an emerging medical technology. Hope is in the heart. It is its own reward. So I would say to those who march with me: Keep the faith, never give up. These are the lessons, the gifts of my miraculous journey, saving Ben.